The Glow of Synthesis

Twelve Beacons of Light in Social Psychiatry

The Glow of Synthesis

Twelve Beacons of Light in Social Psychiatry

Editors

Roy Abraham Kallivayalil
MD DPM
Professor
Department of Psychiatry
Pushpagiri Institute of Medical Sciences, Thiruvalla
Mar Sleeva Medicity
Palai, Kerala, India
Former President, World Association for Social Psychiatry

Rama Rao Gogineni
MD MFT
Professor of Psychiatry and Senior Educator (Developmental Psychiatry)
Cooper Medical School, Rowan University
New Jersey, USA
Former President, American Association for Social Psychiatry

Salman Akhtar
MD ABPN DLFAPA
Emeritus Professor
Department of Psychiatry
Jefferson Medical College
Philadelphia, USA

Foreword

R Srinivasa Murthy

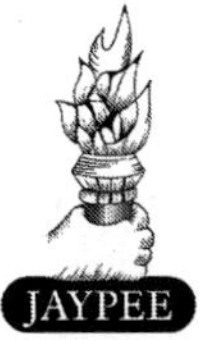

JAYPEE BROTHERS MEDICAL PUBLISHERS
The Health Sciences Publisher
New Delhi | London

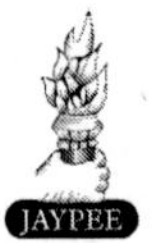

Jaypee Brothers Medical Publishers (P) Ltd

Headquarters
EMCA House
23/23-B, Ansari Road, Daryaganj
New Delhi 110 002, India
Landline: +91-11-23272143, +91-11-23272703
+91-11-23282021, +91-11-23245672
E-mail: jaypee@jaypeebrothers.com

Corporate Office
Jaypee Brothers Medical Publishers (P) Ltd.
4838/24, Ansari Road, Daryaganj
New Delhi 110 002, India
Phone: +91-11-43574357
Fax: +91-11-43574314
E-mail: jaypee@jaypeebrothers.com

Overseas Office
JP Medical Ltd.
83, Victoria Street, London
SW1H 0HW (UK)
Phone: +44-20 3170 8910
E-mail: info@jpmedpub.com

EU GPSR Authorised Representative
Logos Europe, 9 rue Nicolas Poussin
17000, La Rochelle, France
Phone: +33 (0) 6 67 93 73 78
E-mail: Contact@logoseurope.eu

Website: www.jaypeebrothers.com
Website: www.jaypeedigital.com

Inquiries for bulk sales may be solicited at: jaypee@jaypeebrothers.com

The Glow of Synthesis: Twelve Beacons of Light in Social Psychiatry

First Edition: **2025**

Reprint: **2026**

ISBN: 978-93-6616-364-2

Printed at: Samrat Offset Pvt. Ltd.

To

JOSHUA BIERER

(1901–1984)

The first President of the World Association for Social Psychiatry and a tireless proponent of the integral relationship between individuals and their social surround.

Contributors

Andres J Pumariega
MD Board Certified in Psychiatry, Child and Adolescent Psychiatry
Professor and Chief
Division of Child and Adolescent Psychiatry
Department of Psychiatry
University of Florida College of Medicine
Gainesville, Florida, USA

April E Fallon PhD
Clinical Professor
Department of Psychology
Drexel University College of Medicine and Fielding Graduate University
Merion Station PA 19066, USA

Behdad Bozorgnia MD
Psychoanalyst and Psychiatrist
Department of Psychiatry
Perelman School of Medicine at the University of Pennsylvania
Psychoanalytic Center of Philadelphia
Philadelphia, USA

David Ndetei MD FRCPsych
Professor of Psychiatry
University of Nairobi
Nairobi, Kenya

Debasish Basu MD (Psychiatry)
Diplomate of National Board
Professor and Head
Department of Psychiatry
Postgraduate Institute of Medical Education and Research
Chandigarh, India

Fernando Lolas Stepke MD
Professor of Psychiatry
Centro Interdisciplinario de Estudios en Bioética
Universidad de Chile
Diagonal Paraguay 265 - Oficina 806
Santiago de Chile, Chile

Frank Tisano LCSW
Psychoanalyst
Psychoanalytic Center of Philadelphia
Philadelphia, USA

George Christodoulou
MD PhD FICPM FRCPsych
Professor Emeritus
Department of Psychiatry
Athens University
President
European Association of Professors Emeriti
Athens, Greece

George M Gournas
MD PhD CGP ECP Psychiatrist Psychotherapist
Senior Associate
The Athenian Institute of Anthropos (AIA)
Athens, Greece
Member of the AIA Scientific Council

Heather Stuart PhD FRSC CM
Professor and Bell
Canada Mental Health and Anti-stigma Research Chair
Department of Public Health Sciences and Health Services and Policy Research Institute, Queen's University
Kingston, Ontario, Canada K7L 3N6

Juan E Mezzich MD MSc MA PhD
Professor
Psychiatry and of Global Health
Icahn School of Medicine at Mount Sinai, New York

Jyoti M Rao MA LMFT
Faculty
San Francisco Center for Psychoanalysis
San Mateo, CA 94402, USA

Marianne C Kastrup
Specialist in Psychiatry
Former Secretary General
European Psychiatric Association
Copenhagen, Denmark

Mohan Isaac
MBBS DPM MD (Psychiatry) FRCPsych FRANZCP
Clinical Professor of Psychiatry and Consultant Psychiatrist
The University of Western Australia, Perth and Fremantle Hospital
Fremantle, Australia

Rachid Bennegadi MD
Department of Psychiatry
Medical Referent
Sigmund Freud University
Denis, Paris

Rakesh K Chadda
MBBS MD FAMS FRCPsych
Professor and Head
Department of Psychiatry
Amrita Institute of Medical Sciences
Faridabad, India

Rama Rao Gogineni MD MFT
Professor of Psychiatry and Senior Educator (Developmental Psychiatry)
Cooper Medical School, Rowan University
New Jersey, USA
Former President, American Association for Social Psychiatry

Roy A Kallivayalil MD DPM
Professor
Department of Psychiatry
Pushpagiri Institute of Medical Sciences, Thiruvalla
Mar Sleeva Medicity, Palai, Kerala, India
Former President, World Association for Social Psychiatry

Salman Akhtar MD ABPN DLFAPA
Emeritus Professor
Department of Psychiatry
Jeffason Medical College
Philadelphia, USA

Sarah Varun Vas
MD Board Certified in Psychiatry, Child and Adolescent Psychiatry and Addiction Medicine
Clinical Assistant Professor
Department of Psychiatry
University of Florida College of Medicine
Gainesville, Florida, USA

Savita Malhotra MD PhD FRCPsych
President
Indian Psychiatric Society
Former Dean PGIMER, Chandirgarh
Consultant
Fortis Hospital
Mohali, Punjab, India

Tom KJ Craig MBBS PhD FRCPsych
Emeritus Professor of Social Psychiatry
Health Service and Population Research Institute of Psychiatry
Psychology and Neuroscience
King's College
London, UK

Vincenzo Di Nicola
MPhil MD PhD FRCPC FCAHS DLFAPA DFCPA FACPsych
Professor of Psychiatry and Addiction Medicine
Department of Psychiatry and Addiction Medicine
University of Montreal
Montreal University Institute of Mental Health Bureau
Montréal (Québec), Canada

Foreword

*R Srinivasa Murthy**

This book is a very important contribution to Social Psychiatry. The book is published on the 60th Anniversary of the World Association of Social Psychiatry. By compiling the personal lives, contributions of 12+13 pioneers in social psychiatry, both the authors of individual chapters and the editors have done yeoman service to mental health professionals in the field of mental health.

Reading the lives, brought home to me four broad themes: (1) The changes in mental health during the last few centuries; (2) The contributions of the pioneers of social psychiatry; (3) The current mental health challenges and opportunities; (4) A way forward for 'Social Psychiatry'.

Historical Developments in Mental Health Care

The development of the broad field of 'mental health' has been a step-by-step process in the last 5 centuries. Society has come a long way, starting from setting up of 'asylums' for safety of mentally ill persons. The shift from custodial care to humanitarian approach to care (18–19th centuries), the deinstitutionalization movement (20th century) to move mentally ill from asylums to community care (described by Scull as 'asylum as community to community as asylum',[1] to recognition of the rights of persons with mental disorders and the current state of recognition of the importance individuals and the 'live-in' experiences of the persons with mental disorders as important drivers for mental health interventions.[2] At the level of understanding of mental disorders, there are advances—from the period of religious explanations from 'malleus malficorum' of the 15th century, to 'psychoanalysis' of early 20th century, which made the individuals experiences the center of understanding of behavior and behavioral problems, to the current

*Professor R Srinivasa Murthy studied Medicine (1964–1972) at Christian Medical College, Vellore, Tamil Nadu, India. He completed Postgraduate Training in Psychiatry and worked for at Postgraduate Institute of Medical Education and Research, Chandigarh (1972–1981). He was a Faculty Member, The National Institute of Mental Health and Neurosciences (NIMHANS), Bengaluru from 1982–2003 and retired as Professor of Psychiatry. He worked with WHO as a Staff Member from 2000–2001 and 2004–2007. He is currently working on developing and disseminating *Self-care Skills for Emotional Health* for persons living with cancer, their caregivers and caregivers of *Developmental Disabilities.*

understanding based on 'bio-psycho-social-spiritual-environmental' aspects of human behavior. There is a shift from considering persons diagnosed with mental disorders as 'bad', 'mad', or 'sad' towards perception as 'individuals' and as 'equal' members of the society. The recent years of the COVID-19 epidemic has brought to the forefront, the importance of the health of the total population and social determinants of health in general and mental health in particular. The recognition of the health impact of chronic stresses like discrimination and marginalization referred to as 'weathering' calls for societal level interventions.[3] Along with the new understanding, there is a bigger picture of biological aspects of mental health, from thinking of a single molecule like 'dopamine' to 'psychoneuroimmunology'.[4] There have been several important recent international publications namely The Lancet Commission on Mental Health and Sustainable Development of 2018,[5] Lancet-World Psychiatric Association Commission: Time for united action on depression in 2022,[6] the World Mental Health Report, 2022 by the World Health Organization in June 2022,[2] the Lancet Commission on Stigma and Discrimination in October 2022,[7] the Mental State of the World in 2022,[8] the countdown initiative of Global Mental Health Network (GMHN) to monitor the mental health of nations[9] and the Surgeon General Report on 'Our Epidemic of Loneliness and Isolation' released in May 2023[10] and publication of '*The WASP Textbook on Social Psychiatry* in 2023,[11] the book *'Psychiatry in Crisis'* 2021.[12] All these initiatives present a modern view of mental disorders, mental health and well-being which is based on the psychological, social, spiritual and environmental dimensions of mental health.[4]

At a personal level, since the time I entered psychiatry in 1972, I have witnessed a revolution in the way mental health, mental disorders and mental health care are understood and responded to. Let me summarize these changes. In 1972, it was the practice to categorize mental disorders under 'functional psychosis' (to include schizophrenia, manic depressive illness, etc.), and 'organic psychosis'. At that point of time, cognitive disturbances were not recognized as part of functional psychosis or treatment, while in 2023, cognitive aspects of psychosis are a vital part of understanding of all psychosis, as well as interventions. Another example is the identification of 'expressed emotion', in the 1970s. The finding of the family members' reaction to the person with a diagnosis of schizophrenia, as being a vital contributor to the course and outcome of the illness moved the understanding from purely 'psychogenic origin' to the larger psychosocial aspects of life.[13-15] Similarly, advances in psychological therapies like the behavior therapy and cognitive behavior therapy, yoga/meditation, during the last 50 years, created space for the efforts of the individual as an essential part of the therapy. In the last decade, the central role of the individual, in the control of even severe symptoms like hallucinations in the 'Avtar Therapy' has moved the focus back to the individual as the central focus of mental health and well-being.[16] In a dramatic way, the 'deviancy model' that dominated mental health is getting slowly replaced by the 'normalcy model'. At the level of mental health, the recognition of the value of exercise, sleep, nutrition, mindfulness, social connectedness, and spirituality has enlarged the scope of mental health from a purely clinical discipline to one of public health.[17] Similarly emerging issues of loneliness is moving the focus of mental health from illnesses to wellness. A good reflection of these changes is WHO-7 Country Project on *Strategies for Extending Mental Health Care* (1975–1982),[18] and the recent flagship programs like, mental health first aid initiated in Australia in 2001, the initiative of 988 helpline in USA in 2022[19] and the 'Tele-MANAS' program in India in 2022,[20] focusing on 'reaching the unreached' utilizing both the information technology and largely psychosocial interventions at the community level. In a way, public mental health has moved from 'illness to wellness' and 'patients to people'. In all of these developments social psychiatry has been a driving force.

Social Psychiatry Contributions

The detailed personal lives of 12 leaders of social psychiatry and 13 brief biographies illustrate the contributions of these leaders to bring about the changes recounted in the earlier section. Two aspects stand out in the lives of the leaders. Firstly, most of them had lived experiences of persecution, migration, living in different cultures and taking on challenges of the changing society against the backgrounds of the two World Wars and the emerging countries freed from colonial rule. The aspect that impresses me is the way they utilized their experiences to synthesize new ways of understanding human behaviors. **Table 1** summarizes the key contributions of 12 of the pioneers in social psychiatry.

TABLE 1: Key contributions to social psychiatry.

1. Karen Horney, questioned the need and the veracity of these assumptions. Instead of such compulsive and unverifiable reliance upon 'biology', in her view it was better to look for cultural origins of human motivation... Unlike Freud, termed 'the biologist of the mind', Horney became 'the sociologist of the mind'
2. Erich Fromm, felt strongly that to understand what motivates man, one must account for both individual and group dynamics simultaneously, through the lifespan. "Every society has its own distinctive libidinal structure-social dimension of the psyche"
3. Erik Erikson, highlighted the complex interplay of family, culture, and society on human behavior and development, and the need to assess and understand the socioeconomic, interpersonal, and cultural factors that contribute to mental illness
4. Geza Roheim, labeled his cultural theory as ontogenetic, denoting that the developmental experiences of each individual determine the meaning of cultural and social practices and vice versa

Contd...

Contd...

5. Margaret Mead's research stood out from traditional ethnology through its immersive approach, focus on psychological and social processes, cultural relativism, accessibility, and impact...firmly asserted that culture's influence shapes the character, temperament, and personality of individuals within a group
6. Emile Durkheim, empirically demonstrates the variable suicide rates among various social groups to support his theory that the structure of suicide rates is a positive function of the structure of a group or class of people's social relationships and that social relationships vary according to their level of integration and (moral) regulation and suggests that collective public projects will create protective structural changes, more effectively than trying to treat the individual
7. Theodier Adorno, noted that the ultimate source of prejudice has to be sought in social factors which are incomparably stronger than the "psyche" of any one individual involved
8. Joshua Bierer, recognized that 'Mental illness' is an illness, a maladjustment, or a number of states and attitudes, or a combination of several factors... Since social conditions change, each generation has to redefine the meaning of social psychiatry, its relevance and its application to its own social conditions—and not only globally but locally
9. George Carstairs, believed in the importance of social factors in the causation and management of mental disorders
10. Norman Sartorius, assessed the current situation in 2019, about stigma as follows: There are good news and bad news about stigma related to mental illness. The bad news is that stigma is still attached to mental illness and to all that touches it. The good news is that recent years have seen the development of national and regional programs aiming to reduce stigma in many countries
11. Ravi Kapur, disagreed openly with mental health planners who were turning a blind eye to the abundant traditional healing resources available in communities, particularly in rural areas....his experiments with spirituality were also attempts at understanding its role in mental health in the contemporary world
12. Julian Leff, showed experimental evidence for the causal influence for expressed emotions (EE) but also demonstrated the effectiveness of family intervention (FI)

These are only a few of the contributions by the 25 pioneers included in the book.

Current Needs of Mental Health

Four mental health themes face humanity in 2024. Firstly, 'Public mental health' as the future goal of social psychiatry.[12,21,22] Secondly, the recognition of wellbeing as the desired goal of humanity and not only the absence of mental disorders[23-25] and investing in mental health has economic advantages.[26] Thirdly, the recognition of 'Social and Commercial Determinants of Mental Health' as the focus on prevention of mental disorders and promotion of mental health.[27,28] Finally, the growing recognition of the effectiveness interventions using biological (e.g., medicines); psychological (e.g., child rearing, cognitive behavior therapy); social (e.g., addressing inequality, discrimination, social supports, social capital) and spiritual (e.g., surrender, gratitude, forgiveness).[4] Effective interventions are feasible at the levels of individuals, families, communities, larger society, countries and internationally. In a way the visions, dreams and hopes of the pioneers of social psychiatry which form the substance of the book, is getting recognition and showing the paths for action.

However, there are challenges as reflected by the pioneers in different ways in the book.

Carstairs:[29] It seems very likely that in India, in the next generation, we shall see an accelerated disorganization of the old-established sanctions, as the caste system is thrust aside in the process of economic Westernization. Already in the cities of India, there are signs of that dilapidation of social values which Durkheim called anomie: and according to his hypothesis one must predict a great increase in suicide, emotional instability and crime. It will be interesting to see whether this will be borne out, or whether the Indian genius will succeed in adapting itself to the change with less disastrous consequences than the West has shown.

Kleinman: 'What is required is rebalancing of the psychiatric academy to include greater support for researchers conducting social, clinical and community studies?'

Joshua Bierer: 'To take social psychiatry seriously is to take social conditions and social changes seriously and that is why today's social psychiatry is not only Joshua Bierer's social psychiatry and why social psychiatry in Canada is different from its North American neighbor, the USA, and both are very different than the associations in South America like Brazil, and India and Japan in Asia, just to name a few examples.'

Sartorius: 'Emphasizing social factors and social psychiatry was dangerous for one's career in some countries where 'social', 'socialist' and related words were an indication of communist leanings: Senator McCarthy's court cases in the USA and other symptoms of the cold war touched psychiatry as well. Thus, for example, the first meeting of the World Association for Social Psychiatry in London in 1964, was convened at the same time and in the same city as another 'biologically oriented' meeting: colleagues from the West who attended the social psychiatry meeting were not telling others that they attended it. Similarly, but for different reasons, Eastern European psychiatrists were avoiding social psychiatry possibly to remain respected by the majority of psychiatrists in their countries with prevailing biological orientation in psychiatry.'

Leff: Family interventions in schizophrenia: 'Given the influence of NICE and the clear recommendations, it is surprising that family intervention (FI) still struggles to find a home in routine care. Attempts to increase access have included making the training available to NHS professionals including nurses. But sustained uptake is low even in centers where there have been robust efforts to train health staff in the therapy. Barriers to implementation included competing demands of routine work, pressures from delivery of crisis care and significantly a shortage of ongoing supervision after completion of training. In one large mental health center that had been part of this initiative showed a decade later; that fewer than 10% of eligible patients and their families were offered the approach'.

Way Forward

There are challenges to make social psychiatry a reality.

Firstly, though there is recognition of the need to 'empower' the total population with the importance of health in general and mental health in particular, the efforts have been minimal as noted in a recent publication on health literacy.[30] It was observed 'much of the discussion focused on patients and the care team, with only a slight node to communities and health literacy at the population level'. There is an urgent need to move from patients to population and from mental illness to wellness.[4]

Secondly, addressing social/commercial determinants of mental health. As pointed out recently by Beck 'we can no longer fully separate the practice of medicine from politics and policy. Rather, we can come to this intersection with evidence, objectivity, empathy, curiosity, humility, and a dedication to what is right and just'.[31] The mobilization of the policy changes is a task for all stakeholders.

Thirdly, the 'local' nature of the changes that need to be addressed for mental health. The social changes are influenced by historical, cultural, economic and political factors. Social psychiatrists have to develop understandings and interventions that are rooted in the local factors. In addition to bringing about changes, there is need for full utilization of the strengths (e.g., religion/spirituality) of the communities.[32-34]

Fourthly, there is a need for change in the mental attitudes and practices of all mental health professionals. Currently, professionals are more in tune with clinical care and less in public mental interventions. This requires training and reorientation of all professionals.[35,36]

Fifthly, all the changes should be firmly grounded in research evidence and not in ideology and individual opinions. There are specific challenges of availability of tools for measurement of changes and the need for longitudinal studies.

The road ahead is full of challenges and opportunities.

I feel the book will be essential reading for all groups of mental health professionals, planners, media and the general public. I congratulate the authors of the chapters and the editors on this important contribution.

References

1. Scull A. Social order/mental disorder: Anglo American Psychiatry in Historical Perspective. Routledge, London. 1990.
2. World Health Organization. World Mental Health Report: Transforming Mental Health for All. Geneva: World Health Organization, 2022.
3. Geronimus AT. Weathering: the extraordinary stress of ordinary life in an unjust society. Blackstone, 2023.
4. Murthy, R Srinivasa. Concept of Mental disorders, mental health and Well-being. In Meenu Anand (Ed). Mental Health Care Resource Book: concept and praxis for social workers and mental health professionals. Singapore: Springer. 2024. Pp. 25-54.
5. Patel P, Saxena S, Lund C, Thornicroft G, Baingana F, Bolton P et al. The Lancet Commission on Global Mental Health and Sustainable Development. Lancet. 2018;392:1553-98.
6. Herrman H, Patel V, Kieling C, Berk M, Buchweitz C, Cuijpers P, et al. Time for united action on depression: a Lancet—World Psychiatric Association Commission. Lancet, 2022;399:957-1022.
7. Thornicroft G, Sunkel C, Aliev AA, Baker S, Brohan E, El Chammay R, et al. The Lancet Commission on ending stigma and discrimination in mental health. Lancet. 2022;400:1438-80.
8. Thiagarajan T, Newson J. The Mental State of the World in 2022. A publication of the Mental Health Million Project. Sapiens Lab, 2023.
9. United for Global Mental Health. Countdown Global Mental Health 2030. https://unitedgmh.org/knowledge-hub/countd own2030/.
10. Surgeon General. Our Epidemic of Loneliness and Isolation: The US Surgeon General's Advisory on the Healing Effects of Social Connection and Community. Surgeon General. United States of America. Washington. 2023.
11. Gogenini R, Pumariega AJ, Kallivayalil R, Kastrup M, Rothe EM (Eds). The WASP Textbook on Social Psychiatry: Historical, Developmental, Cultural and Clinical Perspectives. Oxford: New York, 2023.
12. Nicola VD, Stoyanov D. Psychiatry in Crisis at the Crossroads of Social Sciences, the Humanities, and Neuroscience. Springer Nature, Switzerland, 2021.
13. Brown GW, Birley JLT, Wing JK. Influence of family life on the course of schizophrenic disorders: a replication. Br J Psychiatry. 1972;121:241-58.
14. Leff J, Wig NN, Ghosh, A. et al. Expressed emotion and schizophrenia in north India. III. Influence of relatives' expressed emotion on the course of schizophrenia in Chandigarh. Br J Psychiatry. 1987;151:166-73.
15. Leff J, Kuipers L, Berkowitz R, et al. A controlled trial of social intervention in the families of schizophrenic patients. Br J Psychiatry. 1982;141:121-34.
16. Garety PA, Edwards CJ, Jafari H, Emsley R, Huckvale M, Rus-Calafell, M. Digital AVATAR therapy for distressing voices in psychosis: the phase 2/3 AVATAR2 trial. Nature Medicine. https://doi.org/10.1038/s41591-024-03252-8.
17. Srinivasa Murthy R. Selfcare for mental health: the new frontier. In G Saha (Ed): different strokes, 2nd edn. Bhopal: Publication of Indian Psychiatric Society, 2016.
18. Murthy R Srinivasa, Wig NN. The WHO collaborative study on strategies for extending mental health care, IV: A training approach to enhancing the availability of mental health manpower in a developing country. American Journal of Psychiatry. 1983;140:1486-90.

19. Miller AB, Oppenheimer CW, Glenn CR, et al. Preliminary Research Priorities for Factors Influencing Individual Outcomes for Users of the US National Suicide Prevention Lifeline. JAMA Psychiatry. 2022;79:1225-31.
20. NIMHANS. Operational Guidelines: The Digital Arm of the National Mental Health Programme, 2022. NIMHANS, Bengaluru.
21. Campion J, Javed A. WPA Working Group on Public Mental Health: objectives and recommended actions. World Psychiatry. 2022;21:330-1.
22. Mehta N, Croudace T, Davies S. Public mental health: evidenced-based priorities. Lancet. 2015; 385(9976):1472-5.
23. Vogt D, Borowski S, Kumar SA, Lee LO, Schnurr PP. Psychosocial well-being at the time of trauma exposure and risk of PTSD. JAMA Netw Open. 2024;7(10):e2440388. doi:10.1001/jamanetworkopen.2024.40388
24. Rottenberg, J, Crispo K. Benefits of Well-Being on Psychopathology—Now for Next Steps. JAMA Network Open. 2024;7(10):e2440331. doi:10.1001/jamanetworkopen.2024.40331
25. Dolan P, Peasgood T, White M. Do we really know what makes us happy? A review of the economic literature on the factors associated with subjective well-being. Journal of Economic Psychology. 2008;29:94-122.
26. Muñoz-Navarro R, Saunders R, Buckman JEJ, Ruiz-Rodríguez P, González-Blanch C, Medrano LA, et al. Investing in mental health: a path to economic growth through psychological therapies. British Journal of Psychiatry. 2024;225:460-1. doi: 10.1192/bjp.2024.70.
27. Gilmore AB, Fabbri A, Baum F, Bertscher A, Bondy K, Chang H, et al. Defining and conceptualising the commercial determinants of health. Lancet. 2023;401:1194-213.
28. Alegría M, NeMoyer, A JD, Falgas I, Wang Y, Alvarez K. Social determinants of mental health: where we are and where we need to go. Curr Psychiatry Rep. 2019;20:95. doi:10.1007/s11920-018-0969-9.
29. Carstairs GM. Attitudes to Death and Suicide in an Indian Cultural Setting. International Journal of Social Psychiatry. 1955;1:33-41.
30. National Academies of Sciences, Engineering and Medicine. Building the case for health literacy: Proceedings of a workshop National Academies Press, Washington, 2018.
31. Beck AF. Election Night. JAMA. Published online November 15, 2024. doi:10.1001/jama.2024.25200.
32. Koenig HG, VanderWeele TJ, Peteet JR. Handbook of Religion and Health, 3rd edn. Oxford: New York, USA, 2024.
33. Murthy R Srinivasa. Integrating spirituality in social work: challenges and opportunities. In: Meenu Anand (Ed). Mental Health Care Resource Book: concept and praxis for social workers and mental health professionals. Singapore: Springer. 2024. Pp. 205-28.
34. Murthy R Srinivasa. Cancer and spirituality: underutilized resource for cancer care in India. Indian Journal of Medical Paediatric Oncology. 2024;45:271-5.
35. Murthy R Srinivasa. Rethinking public mental health: personal reflections. World Soc Psychiatry. 2023;5:106-11.
36. Campion J, Javed A, Saxena S, Sharan P. Public mental health: an opportunity to address implementation failure. Indian J Psychiatry. 2022; 64:113-6.

Preface

All fields of human intellectual endeavor owe their origin to an exceptional individual or a group of such individuals who dared to challenge the stagnancy of knowledge in their era and to forge new and bold pathways for thought, curiosity, and conceptual advancement. Newton in Physics, Darwin in Evolution, Kraepelin in Psychiatry, Freud in Psychoanalysis, Einstein in Science and Mahatma Gandhi in Non-Violent Civic protest are prime examples of such towering figures. The book in your hands is an explication, if not a celebration, of similar geniuses who laid down the foundations of what we have come to know as the subspecialty of social psychiatry.

Social psychiatry is a discipline that focuses on the social dimension of mental health, mental illness, and mental health care. Social psychiatry uses the concepts and methods of social sciences, including psychology, sociology, and anthropology. In 1903, the term "social" was first linked to psychiatry. The First and Second World Wars advanced psychiatry, including social psychiatry. De-colonization, Influenza and COVID-19 epidemics, End of slavery, women's rights, globalization and other significant events highlighted the importance of "social" in understanding and addressing the issues. The tumultuous 1960s brought in the biopsychosocial model. The World Association of Social Psychiatry (WASP) was founded in 1964. We selected 12 main figures and 15 others that contributed a variety of very important, diverse landmark contributions from developmental, bio-psychosocial determinants, and organizational aspects that contributed to current social psychiatry and psychology concepts.

The most powerful element in a personal narrative is the emotional connection one can establish with characters and give to others. We hope these narratives can be used as tools in learning, engaging, for deeper understanding, and love for learning. Our hope is one can make use of these narratives from historical contributors to "social" in psychology and psychiatry to enhance one's knowledge, educate students and trainees, and address biopsychosocial determinants in improving one's functioning and well-being.

Roy Abraham Kallivayalil
Rama Rao Gogineni
Salman Akhtar

Acknowledgment

We are grateful to the National Alliance for Mental Health (NAMH), India, for the support given for the publication of this book.

Contents

PART 1 Culturally Inclined Psychoanalysts

CHAPTER 1

Karen Horney

Salman Akhtar

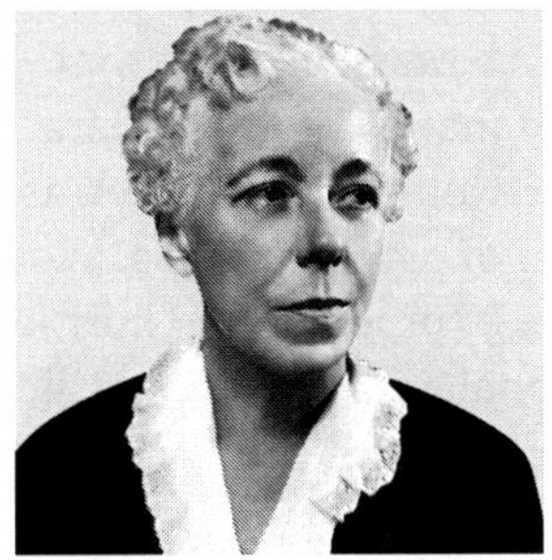

(1885–1952)

INTRODUCTION

A careful scrutiny of the relationship between psychoanalysis and culture reveals a century-long, gradual shift from what I have called "psychoanalytic anthropology" to "anthropological psychoanalysis."[1] The former era (1) regarded culture to be a product of the human mind; (2) mapped personality development in Eurocentric terms; (3) considered an individuated and unitary self to be universal; and (4) barred sociocultural variables from altering the views of psychopathology, treatment, technique, and therapeutic goals. The latter (and the contemporary) era (1) views the human mind as a product of culture; (2) regards personality development as culturally variable; (3) allows for enmeshed and communal selves as also being modal structures; and (4) permits, if not encourages, sociocultural variables to impact upon psychiatric nosology, treatment, technique, and therapeutic goals. Another important difference exists between the early "psychoanalytic anthropology" and the current "anthropological psychoanalysis." The former was the product of heuristic imperialism and deployed psychoanalytic theory in toto in explaining diverse social, historical, political, religious, ethnic, economic, and literary endeavors. The latter gives primacy to the bilateral flow of information between psychoanalysis and other disciplines of the humanities, thus facilitating their dialectical enrichment.

TABLE 1: Notable publications.

- The Neurotic Personality of Our Times (1937)
- New Ways in Psychoanalysis (1939)
- Our Inner Conflicts (1942)
- Neurosis and Human Growth (1950)
- Feminine Psychology: Collected Papers, 1922–137 (1967)

This positive shift has taken many decades, however. Elsewhere,[1] I have elucidated in detail the steps our profession took in this tumultuous journey and the myriad dramatic personae who fomented, fueled, and facilitated this salutary transformation. To be sure, there are many others (e.g., Geza Roheim, Harry Stack Sullivan, Abraham Kardiner, Clara Thompson, Alan Roland, Stuart Twemlow, Dorothy Holmes, and myself as well) who contributed to such cultural rejuvenation of psychoanalysis, a towering early figure among them is that of Karen Horney (pronounced "horn-eye"). This essay is devoted to summarizing her personal and professional life[2-4] as well as the extensive body of her published work **(Table 1)**.

BRIEF BIOGRAPHY

Karen Horney was born as Karen Danielson on September 15, 1885, in the small German town of Eilbeck, near Hamburg. Her father, Brendt Henrik Wackels Danielson, was a Norwegian sea captain who had settled in Germany, and her mother, Cotilde van Ronzelen, was the daughter of an accomplished Dutch architect. Besides the variance in their national origins, Karen's parents had other differences as well. Her father was a Bible-thumping conservative, while her mother was a freethinker. Her father was 20 years older than her mother and "seemed to have no other goal for Karen than having her stay home to help with the housework so that they could dispense with the maid."[2] Her mother, on the other hand, indulged her every wish and stood up for her when, at age 13, Karen announced that she wanted to be a doctor.

After a tumultuous adolescence, Karen moved out of town. She completed her preclinical years at Freiburg University and spent her clinical years at Göttingen and Berlin, graduating from medical school in Berlin in 1913. While still a medical student, in 1909, she married Oscar Horney, who was a budding political economist. A year later, she sought psychoanalytic treatment for depression and sexual difficulties from Karl Abraham (1877–1925), a distinguished analyst and a beloved pupil of the founder of psychoanalysis, Sigmund Freud (1856–1939). Over the next few years, both her parents died; she became a mother and—now known as Karen Horney—joined the Berlin Psychoanalytic Society. Learning from her own life experiences and from her analytic work, which female patients, Horney soon began to write a series of papers that were critical of Freud's patriarchal thrust. She dismissed the centrality of penis envy in female development, asserting that femininity is innate and so is the girl's identification with her mother. Freud was not pleased.

By 1923, Horney's husband began to flounder in his business and also developed meningitis. He grew embittered and argumentative. Their marriage suffered. Horney's only and much-loved older brother's unexpected death at this very time introduced further stress in the marriage. She became depressed and even suicidal but, wisely, sought treatment, this time with the Vienna-born President of the Berlin Psychoanalytic Institute, Hans Sachs (1881–1947). She separated from her husband in 1926 and later got divorced. Her psychoanalytic work flourished, and she published many papers on female psychology.

In 1932, on the invitation of the highly influential psychoanalyst Franz Alexander (1891–1964), Horney moved from Berlin to Chicago. There she helped devise the local institute's training program and taught courses on analytic technique and on female psychology while seeing patients 5 hours a day. She also developed a very active social life, hobnobbing not only with renowned analysts like Karl Meininger (1893–1990) and Lionel Blitzstein (1893–1952) but also sociology's glitterati like Margaret Mead (1901–1978) and Eric Fromm (1900–1980); the latter became her lover. Fascinatingly, Horney's work on feminine masochism also appeared around this time.

Soon she fell out with Alexander, perhaps "because she could not bear being second in command to him."[2] Disenchanted with Alexander and attracted by the iconoclastic interpersonal views of Harry Stack Sullivan (1892–1949) and Clara Thompson (1893–1958), Horney decided to leave Chicago. Being romantically involved with Fromm, who lived in New York, made the choice of her next destination easy.

Horney joined the prestigious New York Psychoanalytic Institute in 1934 and set up home in the wealthy Upper East Side of Manhattan. Fromm remained her constant companion, and their break-up a few years later was bitter and painful. Over time, she bounced back. Her circle of acquaintances grew. The eminent theologian Paul Tillich (1886–1965) became a new friend. Psychoanalysts from the Washington Baltimore Society began to visit her, and she herself commuted to teach at Washington and Baltimore frequently. Her popularity grew, but not so much in the stodgy chambers of classical psychoanalysis. She became well-known among avant-garde psychologists, a teacher in high demand, a "regular" at the recently started New School of Social Research in New York.

She now began to use her own mothering experience to go beyond Freud and replace castration anxiety with the "basic anxiety" of getting or not getting mother's approval. She went on to reject the centrality of the Oedipus complex in the genesis of neuroses and declared that it is maternal neglect and abuse that gives rise to a child's hostility, and this causes guilt and low self-esteem. A child thus afflicted seeks love and protection from father. It is therefore not a biologically fated Oedipus complex but a clingy attachment bred of maternal deprivation that lies at the core of all neuroses. Horney diverged from the traditional Freudians in the matters of therapy as well. She emphasized the importance of focusing upon present realities and fantasies over the reconstruction and interpretation of childhood scenarios. Such disagreements, coupled with her great popularity with educated laity and envy-inducing lavish lifestyle, proved sufficient to make her membership in the New York Psychoanalytic Institute and led to her resignation in 1941.

Soon afterward, she founded the Association for the Advancement of Psychoanalysis and started publishing the American Journal of Psychoanalysis. For the next 7–8 years, Horney remained very active at the psychoanalytic training institute that evolved under the auspices of her association. She lectured, supervised candidates in training, and maintained a private practice of psychotherapy and psychoanalysis. Gradually, she got tired and stopped teaching at both the New School and the American Institute of Psychoanalysis around 1951. In the last year of her life, she found herself increasingly lonely, got in the habit of reading detective stories, and, surprisingly, developed an interest in Zen Buddhism. It is surprising because of the philosophy's insistence upon transcending individuality, while her own work focused upon realizing individuality. Having met a fresh challenge, she visited Japan for a brief period of study in 1952, but soon after coming back from this journey, she was diagnosed to be suffering from cancer. She died at the age of 67 on December 4, 1952, and was buried at the Ferncliff Cemetery in Ardsley, a short distance from New York City.

MAJOR CONTRIBUTIONS

It is hardly possible to summarize a prolific writer and influential theorist's lifelong work in a few pages. The presentation here, therefore, must be considered inherently telegraphic and even incomplete. With this caveat entered, it seems that Horney's contributions can be distilled into the following three categories: (1) Debiologizing human motivation, (2) positing the sociogenesis of emotional disorders, and (3) restoring dignity to female psychology.

Debiologizing Human Motivation

Readers of contemporary psychoanalysis have the benefit of viewing human motivation from the sophisticated prism of object relations theory,[5] attachment theory,[6,7] self-actualization perspective,[8,9] and separation individuation viewpoint.[10] This can lead them to forget that the original psychoanalytic theory was mostly biological in its postulates.

Freud's[11,12] theory of human motivation was based upon "instincts," which he defined as "a concept on the frontier between the mental and the somatic, as the physical representative of the stimuli originating from within the organism, and reaching the mind, and as a measure of the demand made upon the mind for work in consequence of its connection with the body."[12] Freud's[12] first dual instinct theory proposed "sexual" and "self-preservatory" to be the two instincts, but his second dual instinct theory[13] changed this to the formulation of "life instinct" (which subsumed sexual and self-preservatory motives) and "death instinct" (which sought to return the living organism to an inanimate state and whose threat found dilution in being externalized as aggressive drive). Regardless of their reformulation, instincts retained their somatic origins. Their aim "was to find tension relief and their object" was any person (or thing) that facilitated the same.

In this theory, anxiety was caused by the threatening breakthrough of instincts, and defenses were patterned upon the body's aversive responses. Thus, denial was shutting one's eyes, negation was turning one's neck away, introjection was swallowing, projection was spitting, and so on. Phrases such as "oral erotism," "anal sadism," "urethral ambition," "penis envy," and "castration complex" abounded. Relief from bodily tensions was regarded to be the goal of everything people did or wanted to do. The fundamental pressure to act (or, to want to act, to imagine ways of acting) arose from biologically accrued tensions and epigenetic unfolding of preprogrammed, somatic, zonal excitements (e.g., oral, anal, and phallic) that determined the mental preoccupations of the growing human organism. A "sensual current"[14] underlay all motivation, even though its emergence was diphasic: First as polymorphous, partial, and changing pleasures in childhood and next as consolidated genital pleasure in adolescence and adult life. Fixations upon (and regressions to) infantile and childhood zonal expressions manifested as psychopathology; the inadequate advance from the "pleasure principle" to the "reality principle"[15] added to the problem.

Translated into plain English, this implied that the origins of excessive drinking, smoking, incessantly talking, and greedy acquisitiveness resided in an unsatisfactory oral phase; those of orderliness, parsimony, and rigidity were defensive strategies against the dirty pleasures of the anal phase; burning ambition betrayed fixation on the urethral phase; cockiness and exhibitionism emanated from the phallic phase; and so on.

While today's psychoanalysts and psychiatrists correctly regard such reductionism as outdated, the steps away from this kind of thinking was actually taken in Freud's own lifetime by by Alfred Adler[16] and then more forcefully by Karen Horney.[17-20] She questioned the need and the veracity of these assumptions. Instead of such compulsive and unverifiable reliance upon "biology," in her view, it was better to look for cultural origins of human motivation. Do people drink excessively because of an "oral fixation" or in order to relieve feelings of inferiority and incompetence in social situations, for instance? Does the pursuit of enormous wealth betray an anal-retentive pleasure or suggest a vengeful tendency to show off while also depriving others of their due?

Thinking along such lines, Horney delineated 10 basic human needs.[19] These included (1) the need for affection, (2) the need for a partner, (3) the need for recognition, (4) the need for admiration, (5) the need for power, (6) the need for exploitation, (7) the need for achievement, (8) the need for autonomy, (9) the need for perfection, and (10) the need for being inconspicuous. Clearly, some of these leaves were contradictory to others, and such schism, if exaggerated, became one source of neurotic distress. In a later work,[20] Horney condensed these 10 needs into three categories: (1) The need for compliance—this subsumed the first, second, and third needs of the 10 described earlier; (2) the need for expansion—this subsumed needs four through eight; and (3) the need for detachment—this subsumed the former needs nine and 10. Intensifications of these three needs, respectively, produced the tendency to go with people, go against people, and go away from people. This was Horney's foundational "socio-genesis," from which she evolved further refinements and nuances of psychopathology. Unlike Freud, termed "the biologist of the mind" by Sulloway,[21] Horney became "the sociologist of the mind."

Positing Sociogenesis of Psychopathology

In contrast to Freud's emphasis upon the persistence or revivification of infantile psychosexual drives in the causation of neurotic disorders, Horney declared that man's emotional conflicts arose from his struggle with attitudes prevalent in his culture. He described five such attitudes as potential true triggers or second conflicts: "first, attitudes concerning giving and getting attacked affection; second, attitudes concerning evaluation of the self; third, attitudes concerning self-assertion; fourth, aggression; and fifth, fear and sexuality."[18] Horney saw all neurotic suffering as arising from how an individual fails to cope with or becomes unduly compliant to such prevalent expectations of behavior.

Wisely, she cautioned that her portrayal was restricted to her times, and new patterns of neurosis might evolve in the future. Having entered that caveat, Horney delineated the neurotic features that developed in relation to these five cultural attitudes: (1) The need for approval from others grew into indiscriminate hunger for appreciation in the neurotic; (2) the need for an overall positive self-evaluation was defensively transformed in the neurotic feelings of inferiority or remained transparent as convictions "of incompetence, of stupidity of unattractiveness"[18] prevailed; (3) the need for self-assertion was inhibited in the neurotic persons; thus, afflicted could not express their wishes, do things in their own interest, and stand their ground when disputed by others; (4) the need to modulate one's aggression turned uneven, leading the neurotic individual to either becoming domineering and overexacting, or vulnerable to being abused, betrayed, and humiliated; and (5) the need for healthy and pleasurable sexuality ended up as either a compulsive need for sex or inhibitions toward it.

Distinct in Horney's conceptualization of these neurotic syndromes is their etiological linkage to the tension between what is culturally expected of an individual and what he or she is able to accomplish. At the same time, Horney remained mindful of the role of cultural relativism. For instance, she stated that a highly self-effacing and professionally reticent young woman and a laid-back artist who makes little effort to sell his paintings would be considered neurotic in the United States. This judgment would emanate from the culturally shared assumption that everyone should try to get ahead and be economically successful. Horney[18] unmasked the cultural relativism of such "diagnoses" by stating that "if the girl without competitive drives lived in some Pueblo Indian culture, she would be considered entirely normal, or if the artist lived in a village in Southern Italy or Mexico, he, too, would be considered normal, because in these environments, it is inconceivable that anyone should want to earn more money or to make any greater effort than is absolutely necessary to satisfy immediate needs." To be sure, Horney's turn of the 20th century observation seems outdated in today's money-driven world, but the spirit of her assertion lives on: What is neurotic in one culture might be normal in another.

Take, for instance, the following: If a married North American woman in her early 40s calls her mother every day on the phone to seek advice about this or that domestic matter or to simply chat, she is likely to be considered immature, dependent, and insufficiently individuated. However, if a similar woman of an Indian, Bangladeshi, Pakistani, Afghani, Iranian, or Turkish origin (even if she were living as an immigrant in the United States) shows such attachment to her mother, it is unlikely that she would be considered pathological. To wit, our two imaginary women (North American and Asian) might be next-door neighbors, behaving in the exact same manner, with one deemed morbid and the other normal, if not admirable. This cultural relativism is at its zenith, and Horney pointed it out in no uncertain terms.

Going a step further, Horney noted that what is considered normal not only varies with the culture but also within the same culture in the course of time and with different classes of society.[18] No culture is static. Shared patterns of behavior, coping strategies, celebrated and despised group memories, rituals, and forms of social stratification evolve over time. Degrees of sexual freedom, reverence toward authority, and modesty or flashiness of attire are particularly subject to changes from era to era.

When marked, search differences can accentuate customary generational gaps in communication, cause interpersonal strife, and draw attention from mental health professionals. Culture as a given stable structure and as a shifting and changing dynamic both played a central role in Horney's theorizing about the genesis of emotional disorders.[17-20]

Restoring Dignity to Female Psychology

In a series of papers written during the 1920s and 1930s, Horney voiced strong disagreement with Freud's views of girls' psychic development and of women's psychology in general. During their earlier piecemeal appearance, these papers caused little stir, but their collected publication in a single volume[22] with the title Feminine Psychology, during the peak of the feminist movement in the United States and Europe, became a seismic event that shook up the rather darkly monolithic view of female psychology in Freud's writings.

To put it briefly, Freud proposed that, before discovering the anatomical difference between sexes, "the little girl is, it is a little boy,"[23] and after noticing her "organic inferiority,"[24] she developed penis envy and feelings of self-contempt for belonging to "a sex, which is lesser in so important an aspect."[23] Freud talked of the "inferiority of the clitoris"[25] as compared to the penis as a matter of fact. His scheme of female psychosexual development included the girl's repudiation of her lack of penis, anger at the mother for not giving her one, fixating on the clitoris, and developing a "masculinity complex,"[23] reluctantly making an emotional shift from the clitoris to the vagina, and changing the object of her affection from mother to father in the hope of obtaining a penis (or its substitute, a baby) from him. Not subject to castration threat, like boys, girls held on to her Oedipal strivings much longer. All this let them to remain sentimental, lack moral strength and independence, and grow up as individuals with a "lesser sense of justice."[25] If this were not enough, Freud declared that lacking sublimation, women had made few significant contributions to the mankind, with the exception of braid-making (as a penis substitute) and domestication of fire (owing to the prehistoric woman's inability to sit down upon it, urinate, and put it off).

Horney questioned the implicit psychoanalytic view of girls as defective boys and women as frustrated men. According to her, these views had evolved, because the theory was the product of a male mind operating in a male-dominated culture. Horney insisted that females have patterns of psychic development, which are inherently different from males. Drawing upon Horney's 1967 collection of papers on female psychology,[22] Kellman's outstanding survey of her contributions to this realm,[26] and my own careful reading of Horney's work, it seems justifiable to categorize her refinements of psychoanalytic theory vis-à-vis females in the following six areas:

1. *Penis envy:* Horney did not as much refute Freud's concept of penis envy as she questioned its bedrock nature and its purely anatomical explanation. She suggested the penis envy was not ubiquitous and occurred as a metaphorical search for power and admiration only in a male-dominated society. Moreover, the theoretical preoccupation with penis envy detracted from the parallel concept of "womb envy," whereby a male child felt in awe of the mother's capacity to single-handedly bring forth babies in this world (since he knew little about the father's role in procreation). Horney argued that men's pull toward creative work could be seen as a compensation for their small role in making a baby. She concluded that envy was not restricted to girls; children of both sexes envied each other.
2. *The status of the vagina:* Freud[25] proposed that the little girl's focus is upon the clitoris, and her discovery of the vagina is a willy-nilly later developmental step. Horney disagreed. She asserted that the awareness of the vagina, sensations in it, and exploration of it by inserting fingers was evident in little girls from the very beginning. The significance of these observations was to free female psychosexual development from its linkage to a penis-less state and to accord it an independent psychological line of growth and maturation.
3. *Girls wish for a baby:* Contrary to Freud, who had attributed the girl's wish for a baby to her insistent quest for a penis, Horney saw the desire to be primary and hardwired in the female psyche. It reflected a joyous celebration of her body's capacities and a positive identification with a generative mother.
4. *Feminine masochism:* Freud[27] had divided masochism into three types: "primary" (which was the somatic substrate of the death instinct blended with the libido of the life instinct), "erotic" (which was the source of sexually arousing fantasies of being bound, beaten, and humiliated), and "moral" (which emanated from the unconscious guilt and led to chronic self-punishment). Curiously, he used the expression "erotic masochism" interchangeably with "feminine masochism" (even though the two cases from which this idea was derived were both males!). In fact, Freud went on to declare that women possessed an inherently passive and masochistic attitude in both sexuality and in day-to-day life. Horney questioned such generalization and also Freud's conflation of the pathological and normal phenomena. Besides, she felt that social anthropology could shed better light than human anatomy upon the roots of such tendencies in women. A culture's prevalent beliefs, upheld role models, and inherited traditions regarding women were far more responsible for their low self-esteem, submissive attitude, and vulnerability to exploitation and abuse; the latter was mistakenly taken to be their inherent masochism in a patriarchal sleight-of-hand by the medical profession and the public at large.

5. *Women's appearing frightening to men:* Horney stated that that men hide their secret (and, sometimes, not so secret) dread of women by either overidealizing them or by "conquering" and dominating them. Underneath such defensive measures, men remain afraid of women. Horney[22] stated that a woman appears frightening to men "because she holds the secret of life and death; is particularly dangerous when she is menstruating; to deflorate her is most dreadful; and to penetrate her is to chance being castrated."
6. *Women's (apparent) disinterest in sexual intercourse:* Early psychoanalysis attributed women's seeming lack of enthusiasm about penetrative sex to the act being a reminder of her lacking a penis or to the guilt she harbors for wanting her father's penis. Horney considered such speculation to be strangely divorced from the Victorian puritanism in the cradle of which psychoanalysis was born and which looked down upon robustly sexual women. In her view, if a woman displayed disinterest or aversion to sex, it was owing to her internalization and unconscious compliance with the handed-down, erotically disparaging cultural norms.

Putting all these observations together, it is clear that Horney challenged the prudishness of psychoanalysis toward female sexuality and voiced a far more enlightened and libertarian view of women. The fact is that her views profoundly affected later developments in psychoanalysis. Blum,[28] in summarizing these changes, states that "the female super ego is now not regarded as weaker or deficient, and sex differences in the structure and function are not given value judgments. Libido is not masculine, neither are passivity and masochism regarded as essentially feminine traits. Penis envy is no longer considered the bedrock of a woman's disappointment and necessary pronunciation but has been subject to major reinterpretation. Neither masochism not envy is confined to women and are no more necessarily related to the absence of a penis." Instead of a weakness of conscience, one now speaks of a greater relational anchor in moral judgments of women.[29,30] Instead of a femininity that is reluctantly arrived at, there is a celebration of "primary femininity";[31,32] this implies that the girl develops an ego-syntonic (and not an ego-dystonic) mental representation of her genitals from a very early age. Her wish for a baby is no longer reductionistically traced to Oedipal fantasies; it is seen as psychically hardwired and multidetermined. That Karen Horney was the progenitor of these modern ideas goes without saying.

CURRENT STATUS

Horney is well recognized today as one of the earliest and most important "rebels" against Freud's phallocentric and biologically anchored theory of personality development. In the footsteps of Alfred Adler,[16] who had questioned Freud's exclusive focus on sexuality in the origins of neuroses but going many steps farther than him, Horney broadened the reach of psychoanalytic theory to include a vast swath of cultural variables in its developmental schemata, pathogenesis, and therapeutic technique. She downplayed the role of "instincts" and posited that both childhood and adult life anxieties emanate from real and imaginary threats from the interpersonal surround and the culture at large. Seeking approval, love, self-respect, and power are more important determinants of mental health or pathology than the somatic pleasures of the mouth, anus, or genitals. Horney also freed female psychosexual development from the phallocentric shackles of early psychoanalytic theory.

In all these respects, her work enriched that of many other post-Freudian psychoanalysts. The shadow of her description of the need for self-assertion can be discerned in Erikson's[33] ideas on identity. Her concept of "real self" antedated Winnicott's[8] proposal of "true self." Her interest in self-expression, assertiveness, and power has echoes in the self-psychological writings of Kohut.[9] And, according to Paris,[3] "Alice Miller's discussion of the loss and search of the true self in childhood often sounds like Karen Horney, as does R.D. Laing's account of ontological insecurity (which is comparable to her "basic anxiety") and the development of a false system in response to it."

Despite such pervasive influence, Horney's name has lost some of its original luster, and she has become more of a relic. This is because what she had so boldly proposed in the 1920s and 1930s (and what was widely celebrated in the 1960s) has now become all too accepted and commonplace in psychoanalytic theory and practice. One exceptional area in which her name is still taken with great admiration and respect, however, is in female psychology. Knighted as one of the "Mothers of Psychoanalysis,"[2] Horney figures prominently in the pantheon of the feminist critique of psychoanalysis. Her work has gone a long way in rescuing women from the caricatured and devalued portrayal in psychoanalysis, and the impact of her corrective assertions reverberates centripetally to general psychiatry as well, where terms such as "hysterical" and "female masochism" have been relegated to the dustbin of history. The Association for the Advancement of Psychoanalysis that Horney had founded in 1941 and the American Institute of Psychoanalysis, which emerged some years later in New York, continue to flourish even now. The association's flagship journal, The American Journal of Psychoanalysis, has continued publication over the last 80 years, and under the current editorship of the New York-based Hungarian emigre psychoanalyst, Giselle Galdi, is considered one of the topmost avenues of expression in the field.

CONCLUDING REMARKS

Karen Horney was an early psychoanalyst of German origin who migrated to the United States in the early 1930s. She published many important works and, alongside Harry Stack Sullivan, Clara Thompson, and Eric Fromm, came to represent the Neo-Freudian school of psychoanalysis. The main thrust of her contributions was to replace Freud's biological orientation with the role of cultural forces in personality development and in the causation of psychopathology. She questioned Freud's biased and negative portrayal of female psychology and established a line of female psychic development independent of its male counterpart. With regard to psychotherapeutic technique, Horney recognized that addressing childhood conflicts was essential but placed greater importance upon the anxieties experienced by patients in their current lives, especially the tensions derived from their trying to (or failing to) live up to the normative expectations of their culture. For her, "there and then" paled in comparison to "here and now." In other words, the reconstruction of childhood trauma was less significant than the elucidation of current interpersonal anxieties. Horney's perspective was culturally anchored, gender-attuned, and open to both the old and new, the well-established, and yet to be discovered.

While covering a wide-ranging terrain of Horney's biography, theoretical innovations, and professional disputes, this discourse seems incomplete and peculiarly unsatisfying without shedding further light on two major milestones in her life. These nodal points involved her becoming a culturally focused theorist and her radical break from mainstream psychoanalysis in the last decade of her life. Following Horney's own lead, we can see that environmental factors played a significant role in both these developments.

Having been raised by two immigrant parents from two different countries in a seaport community of a third country most likely had sensitized young Karen to the importance of culture in day-to-day life. The facts that (1) her parents differed sharply in their degree of religiosity, (2) she undertook many long journeys with her seafaring father, (3) she was discouraged by him in becoming a physician, because she was a girl, (4) she married a man with a different ethnic background than both her parents, (5) she divorced when it was uncommon to do so, and (6) she migrated from Germany to the United States—all contributed to her astute cultural sense, affirming, in a circular fashion, her assertion that culture (far more than biology) is responsible for the vicissitudes of one's life.

Horney's disengagement from mainstream psychoanalysis also seems culturally determined. Surrounded by married, Jewish, Freud-worshiping, American and East European emigre male psychoanalysts, Horney, a divorced, Freud-refuting, Christian woman of Scandinavian ancestry, could hardly sustain her welcome. She had to leave. Culture, the cornerstone of her life's work, did not prove to be her ally in this decisive turn of events. Paradoxically, though, this proved the very point she had been forcefully making via her theoretical contributions: culture matters!

REFERENCES

1. Akhtar S. Mind, Culture, and Global Unrest. London: Karnac Books; 2018.
2. Sayers J. Mothers of Psychoanalysis. New York: W.W. Norton; 1993.
3. Paris B. Karen Horney. In: Levin E (Ed.). The Freud Encyclopedia. New York: Routledge; 2002. pp. 261-4.
4. Galdi G. Celebrating the 75th anniversary of the American Journal of Psychoanalysis. Am J Psychoanal. 2015;75(1):1-2.
5. Fairbairn WRD. An Object Relations Theory of Psychoanalysis. New York: Basic Books; 1952b.
6. Bowlby J. Attachment and Loss, Vol I: Attachment. New York: Basic Books; 1969.
7. Bowlby J. Attachment and Loss, Volume II: Separation. New York: Basic Books; 1973.
8. Winnicott DW. Maturational Processes and the Facilitating Environment. New York: International Universities Press; 1965.
9. Kohut H. Restoration of the Self. New York: International Universities Press; 1977.
10. Mahler MS, Pine F, Bergman A. The Psychological Birth of the Human Infant. New York: Basic Books; 1975.
11. Freud S. Three essays on the theory of sexuality. Standard Edition of the Complete Psychological Works of Sigmund Freud. London: Hogarth Press; 1905. pp. 123-246.
12. Freud S. Instincts and their vicissitudes. Standard Edition of the Complete Psychological Works of Sigmund Freud. London: Hogarth Press; 1915. pp. 117-40.
13. Freud S. Beyond the pleasure principle. Standard Edition of the Complete Psychological Works of Sigmund Freud. London: Hogarth Press; 1920. pp. 7-64.
14. Freud S. Formulations on the two principles of mental functioning. Standard Edition of the Complete Psychological Works of Sigmund Freud. London: Hogarth Press; 1911. pp. 213-26.
15. Freud S. On the universal tendency to debasement in the sphere of love Contributions to the psychology of love, II. Standard Edition of the Complete Psychological Works of Sigmund Freud. London: Hogarth Press; 1912. pp. 178-90.
16. Adler A. The Practice and Theory of Individual Psychology. Berlin: Verlag Press; 1924.
17. Horney K. The Neurotic Personality of our Time. New York: W.W. Norton; 1937.
18. Horney K. New Ways in Psychoanalysis. New York: W.W. Norton; 1939.
19. Horney K. Our Inner Conflicts. New York: W.W. Norton; 1942.
20. Horney K. Neurosis and Human Growth. New York: W.W. Norton; 1950.
21. Sulloway F. Freud: Biologist of the Mind. Cambridge: Harvard University Press; 1992.
22. Horney K. Feminine Psychology: Collected Papers—1922-1927. New York: W.W. Norton; 1967.
23. Freud S. New introductory lectures on psychoanalysis. Standard Edition of the Complete Psychological Works of Sigmund Freud. London: Hogarth Press; 1933. pp. 7-182.
24. Freud S. Female sexuality. Standard Edition of the Complete Psychological Works of Sigmund Freud. London: Hogarth Press; 1931. pp. 223-43.

25. Freud S. Some psychical consequences of the anatomic distinction between the sexes. Standard Edition of the Complete Psychological Works of Sigmund Freud. London: Hogarth Press; 1925. pp. 241-58.
26. Kelman H. Karen Horney on female psychology. Am J Psychoanal. 1967;27(2): 163-83.
27. Freud S. The economic problem of masochism. Standard Edition of the Complete Psychological Works of Sigmund Freud. London: Hogarth Press; 1924. pp. 157-70.
28. Blum H. Female psychology in progress. J Am Psychoanal Assoc. 1996;44:3-9.
29. Bernstein D. The female superego: a different perspective. Internat J Psychoanal. 1983;64:187-200.
30. Gilligan C. In a Different Voice: Psychological Theory and Women's Development. Cambridge, MA: Harvard University Press; 1982.
31. Stoller RJ. Primary femininity. J Am Psychoanal Assoc. 1976;24(Suppl.):59-79.
32. Kulish N. Primary femininity: clinical advances and theoretical ambiguities. J Am Psychoanal Assoc. 2000;48:1355-79.
33. Erikson EH. Childhood and Society. New York, NY: W.W. Norton; 1950.

Erich Fromm

Frank Tisano

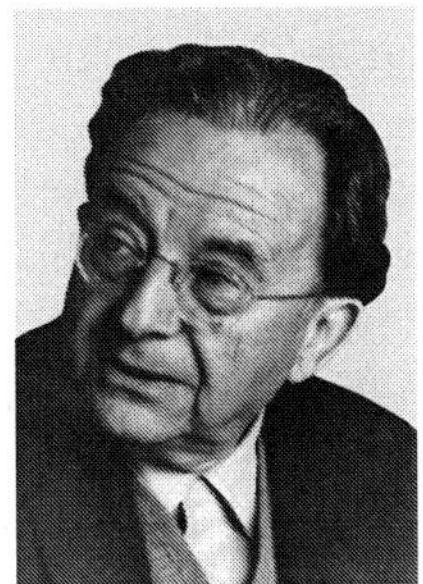

(1900–1980)

INTRODUCTION

Erich Fromm holds a unique place in the field of psychoanalysis and psychiatry. As McLaughlin put it, "Fromm has the distinction of having been central to, but then essentially purged from, the early history of both the Frankfurt School of critical theory and Freudian thought in America."[1] Fromm had an unbelievable knack for identifying and associating with the intellectual heavyweights of his time: Martin Buber, Franz Alexander, Theodore Reik, Karen Horney, Theodore Adorno, Wilhelm Reich, Harry Stack Sullivan, William Fullbright, among others.[2] His writing straddles psychology, sociology, theology, economics, philosophy, politics, anthropology, and history. His remarkable synthetic abilities led him to fuse and harmonize various disciplines. He was a fleet-footed intellectual, and he wrote in a pleasing and persuasive style that garnered mass appeal. Like many of his generation, his life was torn apart by World War II. He fled to the United States, suffered devastating personal losses, and immersed himself in the causes and nature of monumental human destructiveness. Though some have called his personality strident and authoritarian,[3] Fromm also embodied his own injunction to overcome personal and professional alienation, to seek truth no matter how unpopular. At various times, Fromm led a communal group treatment facility, started a low-fee clinic, performed large clinical trials, taught at universities and psychoanalytic institutes, practiced psychoanalysis, advised national leaders, and wrote continuously throughout his life **(Table 1)**.

TABLE 1: Notable publications.

- Escape from Freedom (1941)
- Man for Himself (1947)
- The Sane Society (1955)
- The Art of Loving (1956)
- Marx's Concept of Man (1961)
- The Anatomy of Human Destructiveness (1973)
- To Have or To Be? (1976)

BRIEF BIOGRAPHY

Erich Fromm was born on March 23, 1900, in Frankfurt am Main, Germany. He was the only child to Rosa and Naphtali and was raised in an Orthodox Jewish home. Fromm saw his father as ineffectual, his mother smothering, and their marriage strained, which produced in him an "unbearable, neurotic child."[3] During his youth, he developed what would be a lifelong appreciation for the mystical Hasidic tradition, which emphasized feeling and meditation over economic pursuits.[3] He took private lessons with Salman Rabinkov at 12, moral instruction that he drew from for his whole life thereafter. He admired his uncle Emmanual, which led him to university to study law. Fromm did this for only two semesters before transferring to pursue graduate work in sociology. His personal and scholarly interest in Jewish thought brought him into the orbit of influential theologian Martin Buber.[4]

Fromm started an analysis with Frieda Reichmann, which spilled into an affair and later marriage. Reichmann, over a decade Fromm's senior, was a brilliant thinker in her own right. Together they created a quasi-utopian therapeutic facility for the mentally ill, where they lived with patients in a kibbutz-style homestead, with traditional Jewish meals and rituals. Reichmann introduced Fromm to psychoanalysis, connecting him to psychoanalytic training, which was to be an enduring intellectual pursuit for Fromm, although their marriage was short-lived. Along with a handful of other analysts, including Otto Fenichel and Wilhelm Reich, Fromm became interested in the revolutionary potential of combining individual and social theories, most especially Marx with Freud.[4]

Fromm deepened his ties to psychoanalytic social theory by joining the Frankfurt School, of which he was a key early member. There, he participated in the fruitful explosion of ideas, such as launching a study of German working-class attitudes about authority and conformity. His relationship with the institute soured over an increasingly wide gulf between his and their social and psychological theories. Fromm engaged in a spirited, written debate with Herbert Marcuse, in which Marcuse broadly accused Fromm of diluting Freud's radical mission by abandoning instinct theory. At the time, Marcuse was seen to have trounced Fromm, but by today's standards, there has been a reversal: Fromm (not Marcuse) was the iconoclast! It was he who was putting forth ideas intolerable to the Freudian orthodoxy of his day.

Fromm and Reichmann continued to be married long after the relationship fizzled; indeed, Fromm was likely still married to Reichmann when he transferred his romantic devotion to another towering psychoanalyst of the day, Karen Horney. Fromm and Horney fled Europe during the Second World War. Fromm was active in lobbying for friends and relatives to find safe passage out of Nazi territories and spent large sums to finance their escape. Nevertheless, Fromm suffered many family deaths due to the camps. Fromm's direct, traumatic experience with the rise of Nazism provided ample philosophical inspiration, culminating in his magnum opus on the theory of authoritarianism, *Escape from Freedom*, published in 1941, which launched his career as a public writer and intellectual. Through and with Horney, Fromm leapt into another radical and explosive coterie of thinkers, this time in New York. At Columbia University, Fromm met Harry Stack Sullivan and became integral to the establishment of the William Alanson White Institute.

At age 43, Fromm married Henni Gurland, who suffered from health problems and major depressive episodes. In 1950, hoping that a warm atmosphere would have salutary effects on Henni, the family moved to Mexico City. There, Fromm helped establish the psychoanalytic training program at the national university. Fromm was (and continues to be) a leading thinker in Mexican psychoanalysis. During his 23 years in Mexico, Fromm became enamored of Zen meditation and struck up a correspondence with D.T. Suzuki. Henni died by suicide in 1950. A year later, Fromm married Annis Freeman, with whom he remained loyal until his death. Fromm's passionate, enduring love for Annis provided the direct experience to germinate Fromm's best-known work, *The Art of Loving*.[5]

Trained both as a sociologist and a psychoanalyst, Fromm existed at the intersection of the psyche and the social. In later life, though, he became increasingly connected with American policymakers and politicians. He became a true public intellectual, appearing on national talk shows and establishing correspondences with leading figures such as Adlai Stevenson and William Fulbright, who sought his counsel on complex foreign affairs topics such as nuclear disarmament. Fromm spent his final years in Switzerland, where he remained active both as a psychoanalyst and a writer. He died in Muralto, Switzerland, March 18, 1908, at the age of 79 years.

MAJOR CONTRIBUTIONS

Fromm was a prolific writer whose work spans vast topics, historical eras, and fields of study. Fromm's intellectual magpie nature and disregard for traditional academic lanes were both his genius and his struggle, because he rarely fit neatly in any professional home. Indeed, Fromm would have had it no other way. Fromm believed that productivity came from the seeking of wholeness and truth, and specialization alienated people from their full potentialities. Indeed, some[1,6] argue that it was his "optimal marginality" that gave him psychological freedom to accomplish what he did. Fromm's best-known publications are written in gorgeous, lucid English prose, despite his being a native German speaker. Fromm is best known for his books *Escape from Freedom*[7] and *The Art of Loving*.[5] Both offer trenchant, sweeping observations on some of the thorniest areas of human life: The nature of love, the concept of social character, and thoughts on freedom and authoritarianism.

The Nature of Love

Fromm's *The Art of Loving* offers a comprehensive survey of love in its multifaceted incarnations. Fromm details different kinds and qualities of love, what is psychologically required to love, why we need love, popular misconceptions about love, and the social pressures that facilitate and impede love. Fromm diverged from Freud in his basic assumptions about human nature. Fromm believed, like the interpersonal thinkers of his day (and later the relational school), that people were not principally motivated by instincts. Freud's instinct-dominated view of human nature can be summarized as follows: "We may therefore well conclude that instincts and not external stimuli are the true motive forces behind the advances that have led the nervous system, with its unlimited capacities, to its present high level of development."[8] Fromm followed the insights of anthropologists of his era, who contended that the human has evolved beyond all other mammals in our ability to transcend instinctual nature. Fromm believed that all people have a terror of aloneness, an insight that anticipated (and was later confirmed by) attachment studies.[9] People seek connection at all costs, and therefore, a primary life mission is to "leave the prison of his aloneness".[5] "This need to be at one with others is his strongest passion, stronger than sex and often even stronger than his wish to live."[10] Freed as we are from the shackles of instinct, people are wildly divergent in our life missions, making us far more reliant than other mammals on the often fickle, changing tides of culture to succeed in bonding and reproduction, leading us to want what does not lead to happiness or well-being.

In this regard, Fromm is highly critical of modern culture. As a consequence, Fromm believed that love "is one of the most basic needs of man" but tragically, "I would say that love today is a relatively rare phenomenon" (Interview with Mike Wallace, CBS News, 5/25/1958).[11] Fromm felt that the West was fixated on love but was not especially good at helping people to learn how to love. He argued the abundance of sentimental symbols and tropes around love in Western society reveals our vacuousness, a "symptom of inward emptiness."[12]

Fromm regarded love as a developmental achievement. One of the primary missions of psychoanalysis is to help a patient learn how to love. Fromm and Freud found agreement here. Their paths diverged, however, as to the source of the inability to love. Freud[13] attributes the impediment to an unresolved Oedipal complex. Fromm places greater emphasis on overcoming one's narcissism and counter-dependency. To Fromm, humans are by nature dependent on others from the moment of birth onward. Finding a partner is an admission that we are better together than apart, and therefore, the other person has something I cannot give myself. To Fromm, there are very common barriers to intimacy that must be resolved before successful loving is accomplished: "Psychoanalytic studies show that sexual problems are usually caused not by physical defects nor by lack of knowledge of right techniques, but by psychological inhibitions which make love impossible. Fear or hostility toward the opposite sex prevents persons from living themselves completely, from acting spontaneously, from trusting the sexual partner in the intimacy of physical closeness."[12]

A common misconception is that people believe that they need only to "find" love. Placing the emphasis on the love that is missing "out there" is to miss the point, according to Fromm, because it neglects entirely the process of developing one's own capacity to love. Fromm recommended our society refocus our energies toward the active stance of "loving" rather than "being loved." Love is a capacity that can be actively grown and developed, like other lines of development. Moreover, this stance emphasizes the role of action in love. One cannot love that which he does not tend to. Of this, Fromm quips, "If a woman told us that she loved flowers, and we saw that she forgot to water them, we would not believe in her 'love of flowers.'"[5] It is precisely through the devotion and active concern for those we love that one experiences and expresses love.

Fromm contends that love can be found in both maternal and paternal forms, both necessary to facilitate health and development.[3] Maternal love is a love that conveys you are loveable as you are, life is good, and worth living. Paternal love is contingent and demands the meeting of life's challenges to maintain this love. In this, through the tension of self-acceptance and the need for growth—the paradox of being enough while imagining a future self that is more whole, that balances the scales of living.

Finally, Fromm rejected the premise that individual love relationships are the highest and most natural form of love. Fromm believed that loving a romantic partner was a useful concentration of one's loving energy, but it is only one component of human love. At its best, individual love, for Fromm, was a vessel to launch the individual toward love of all people. Fromm went so far as to say that individual love could not be cleaved from the love of humanity. And it is commonly the case that individual love serves the defensive purpose of shielding oneself from the grander and deeper love of humans, writ large.

The Concept of "Social Character"

Fromm lamented that sociology and psychoanalysis had not been adequately put into conversation with one another.[14] Freud wrote persuasively about social matters, as in *Civilization and its Discontents*[15] and *Group Psychology and the Analysis of the Ego*,[16] but he did not weave these back into his model of the mind. Indeed, in *Civilization*, Freud claims, "originally the ego includes everything, later it separates off an external world from itself."[15] Fromm felt strongly that to understand what motivates man, one must account for both individual and group dynamics simultaneously through the lifespan. The concept of "Social Character" is Fromm's elegant answer to this perceived deficiency. Since Fromm believed that man's greatest fear was aloneness and isolation, he contended that man is highly, perhaps singularly motivated to belong in the world around him. Fromm marveled at the extraordinary malleability of human beings, who are capable "to adapt to almost any conceivable condition of life."[7] This has a tremendous evolutionary advantage. The earliest and the most profound way that culture is transmitted is via parent to child, for "the average family is the 'psychic agency' of society."[17] In this way, the child takes in what will be essential to thrive in the next iteration of human culture. The function of both formal and informal education is "to mold his character in such a way that it approximates the social character, that his desires coincide with the necessities of his social role."[7] Naturally, adaptation to life in the Amazonian jungle will differ from life among the skyscrapers of Manhattan. By analyzing various cultural configurations, Fromm threaded together a theory of how "specific cultures created specific 'configurations' of self, society, and emotionality..."[3] Therefore, the social shapes the man, including shaping his desires toward what is culturally useful: "By adapting himself to social conditions man develops those traits that make him desire to act as he has to act."[7]

Just as we might apply a character type to a patient, Fromm says cultures at large can be distilled around a selection of traits that are dominant, valued, and rewarded. To isolate one such culture, we might think of ancient Greece and note the emphasis on valor and courage in war as a primary element of their social character. To be brave in battle was highly valued, a marker of good character, and helped orient a young person toward a viable life path. The extent to which the individual molds oneself in the direction of what is valued during their time and place goes a long way to determine their success. Therefore, Fromm defines social character thusly: "The social character comprises only a selection of traits, the essential nucleus of the character structure of most members of a basic group which has developed as the result of the basic experiences and mode of life common to that group."[7]

To Fromm, people who are basically in harmony with the social character of their group are said to have productive characters. Fromm believed, like Marx, that the basic position of the human animal is "movement."[18] Therefore, the productive organism is able to continue moving and growing, which leads to a personal sense of well-being, while the unproductive person fails to grow, stagnates, and suffers. As such, humans have an instinctual push toward growth but are not principally motivated by the mechanistic discharge of instincts, as Freud suggested. Rather, our instincts facilitate a push to achieve social purposes, purposes that are ends in themselves.

People who are in disharmony with the prevailing social character, who fail to thrive in their culture, form unproductive characters, of which Fromm describes several subtypes, including the passive-receptive, hoarding, marketing, and exploitative personalities. Fromm believed that these character types could apply to individuals, but also certain epochs and cultural configurations will select for certain unproductive character types. For example, in advanced capitalist economies, we find hoarding to be a dominant form of unproductive character. Or, as Funk has put it, "Thus 'every society has its own distinctive libidinal structure' (Fromm, 1932), which can be studied by looking at the libidinal structure which causes large numbers of individuals to think, feel and act similarly."[19]

Fromm believed that social character was a neutral phenomenon, which could have a salutary or harmful effect on the individual, depending entirely on how well the society is functioning. In other words, individual health is highly correlated with the health of the society. This, Fromm believed, was a major omission from classical psychoanalytic thinking. Fromm argues: "Most psychiatrists take the structure of their own society so much for granted that to them that the person who is not well adapted assumes the stigma of being less valuable."[7]

This raises the unsettling question of what happens to individuals when their society is functioning poorly. Fromm stated the conundrum thusly: "Is an individual sane when he or she is adjusted to an insane society?"[20] Fromm offers a definitive answer: No: "A healthy mind—with exceptions of course—can exist only in healthy societies, and that therefore the problem of individual mental health and social mental health simply cannot be separated for mankind."[20]

Fromm was concerned about two undertheorized, undesirable outcomes: The healthy person who becomes unwell in an unhealthy society and the unhealthy person in sync with the unhealthy society, who is asymptomatic and therefore appears healthy but is not.[21] Fromm coined the term "socially patterned defect" to refer to this second category—the ostensibly healthy person who has adapted well to an insane society.[22] In contrast to Freud's concept of neurosis, Fromm describes the suffering of alienation that is externally generated.

Fromm was deeply troubled by the coercive, culturally imposed pressure to conform to "normalcy." As Funk points out, the "productive or non-productive quality can differ between the individual and the social character, so that an inner psychic conflict arises between the orientations of the two character formation processes and can bring about illness as a result."[19]

To address the problem of the socially patterned defect and alienation due to flawed social character, Fromm proposed an alternate definition of mental health on the basis of humanistic ideals: "The humanistic concept of mental health is an entirely different one. It is one in which mental health is not determined by the proper functioning in any given society but is determined by criteria that are inherent in humankind."[20]

Thoughts on Freedom and Authoritarianism

With both personal and philosophical motivations, Fromm was eager to explain how an advanced industrial nation, such as Germany, brimming with talented intellectuals and a highly sophisticated cultural tradition (music, painting, literature, and science), could descend so rapidly into malevolent authoritarianism.

In his masterful *Escape from Freedom*,[7] Fromm grounds his analysis in historical, economic, and political conditions. Fromm engages the question of how exactly life changed for the average person in Europe from the medieval period to present-day life under capitalism. Fromm believed that fundamental changes in the structure of society would dramatically alter the existential position of the individual in that society. The modified existential position of the individual would, in turn, reshape the political structure in accordance with new psychological needs and demands.

For Fromm, the axis on which everything hinged was freedom: "What characterizes medieval in contrast to modern society is its lack of individual freedom."[7] Generally speaking, one was born into a particular class and performed the occupational functions of that class. The social role was relatively fixed and clear. This was a stable system, because one's psychological well-being was tethered to one's religious life. Earthly conditions were subordinate to the condition of one's soul, which would be measured upon judgment after death. To Fromm, this social model offered a form of psychic stability that is practically unimaginable to the modern reader.

Fromm argued that the protestant reformation was central to dismantling the medieval system, pushing society in the direction of individual liberty. This paved the way for enlightenment thinking and a society that was more tolerant of economic gain, surplus, and social mobility. While the advantages to individual freedom are abundant (e.g., greater ability to choose what to believe, what to strive for, what to do for work and play, and who to love), there are massive hidden costs. Fromm argued that loss of religious orientation and increased personal choice had the unintended outcome of making people more anxious, uncertain, and alone. By removing the stability of medieval life, but without offering clear pathways to fulfillment, Fromm maintains that people reacted by hastily abdicating their newly won freedom: "We have been compelled to recognize that millions in Germany were as eager to surrender their freedom as their fathers were to fight for it;

that instead of wanting freedom, they sought for ways of escape from it; that other millions were indifferent and did not believe the defense of freedom to be worth fighting and dying for."[7]

The regressive desire to relinquish one's individual freedom under capitalism is what Fromm means by the "Escape from Freedom." Fromm attributes the escape from freedom as kindling, the key phenomenon, to understand the rise of authoritarian regimes such as that of Nazi Germany. This boomerang back into tyranny and collapse of individual freedom is the "out of the frying pan, into the fire" problem of modern life. In this context, "The frightened individual seeks for somebody or something to tie his self to; he cannot bear to be his own individual self any longer, and he tries frantically to get rid of it and to feel security again by the elimination of this burden: the self."[7] In summary, individual freedom is de facto good but only insofar as one is able to mobilize that freedom productively. When a society fails to provide the conditions for appropriate utilization of individual freedom, the population is poised to respond by abandoning their freedom, often surrendering their hard-won freedom to an undeserving leader.

Related to the question of freedom is the problem of human destructiveness. Fromm proposed a modified version of Freud's[23] concept of life and death drives, framing human potential in terms of biophilia and necrophilia. When humans are frustrated in their ability to be productive, they become destructive: "The more the drive toward life is realized, the less is the strength of destructiveness. Destructiveness is the outcome of an unlived life."[7] Authoritarian society, therefore, is a natural outgrowth of mass production of unlived lives, who are then motivated to hitch their wagon to a powerful leader that will amplify the destructive potential inside individuals: "Human destructiveness is not caused by animal inheritance but by the existential condition of man, which I'm under certain conditions results in destructiveness and cruelty much greater than that of any animal on the basis of instincts."[3]

CURRENT STATUS

Fromm studies are experiencing a renaissance. Despite the massive popularity of his writings to the general public, Fromm never really achieved a foothold in psychoanalytic circles in America or Europe. His stature diminished precipitously after the public spat with Marcuse and never fully recovered. But societal changes and the evolution of the field have led to a positive reappraisal of Fromm's work, as evidenced by a recent issue of *Psychoanalytic Inquiry* entirely dedicated to Fromm. This year (2024) also marks the announcement of an inaugural Fromm Conference put on by the Erich Fromm Society of North America. Why, after years mired in psychoanalytic obscurity, is Fromm being resurrected now? If we were to pose this question to Fromm himself, we can imagine him answering the way he did in *Escape from Freedom*: "Ideas can become powerful forces, but only to the extent to which they are answers to specific human needs prominent in a given social character."[7] In other words, his ideas have bubbled back to the surface precisely because of the conditions of our present life.

One reason Fromm's ideas resonate now is that his thinking accounts for the social dimension of the psyche, which has become an object of intense theorizing in the last decade. This was a major oversight, which has led to more sophisticated understandings of social identities and the way they interact in the group context. As Frie points out, we need a deep exploration of human nature that includes the social dimension of the psyche to address hyper-relevant questions such as: How ought an analyst comport oneself in a "systemically oppressive" society?[24]

Furthermore, in contrast to the baby boomers, younger generations have grown up in a world of recession, pandemic, exponentially growing college costs, and looming climate catastrophe. For many, there is pessimism about the ability to do as well (let alone better) than one's parents, and doubt that hard work will lead to prosperity. In such a context, there is an appetite to understand what precisely happened to our society. And why can I not thrive in the way that generations did before me? Fromm does offer reassurance to the alienated and marginal among us. He said, in essence, our society is not normal. So, if it is not working for you, that is not so surprising. Needless to say, one can also err in the opposite direction by defensively rationalizing one's problems as socially generated and refusing to acknowledge aspects of life where one does have agency and the ability to grow.

One of the most important innovations of Fromm is his recommendation to critically examine one's present society rather than assuming that it is "sane" and "normal." Indeed, Fromm offered prescient insights about America and life under capitalism, many of which still apply, some more now than ever.[25] Here is a selection of insights Fromm offers to help us look critically at our present condition: (1) Accelerating alienation of capitalism; (2) global rise in authoritarianism (as both symptom and cause of systemic problems); and (3) metastasizing of marketing personalities and aloneness in our technological age.[26]

1. Capitalism produces societal values that are assumed to be universal but are, in fact, a reflection of the current social order. As Friedman[3] writes, in the prototypical capitalist social character, "discipline, thrift, deferred gratification and duty became dominant traits...while sensuality, pleasure, enjoyment, kindness, empathy, sharing, and love came to be devalued." Our society is, to Fromm, excessively competitive, rational, materialistic, and work-oriented: "As a result of this materialism, I think we are getting more and more dehumanized—not in the sense of cruelty but in the sense of losing respect for individuality, for love, for all of the specifically human qualities which have been the content of our religious

and humanistic traditions."[27] We have become dependent on the market economy, which transforms people into objects of money-making and advertisement: "Evidently this type of thinking has a profound effect on our educational system. From grade school to graduate school, the aim of learning is to gather as much information as possible that is mainly useful for the purposes of the market. Students are supposed to learn so many things that they have hardly time and energy left to think."[17] The scientific and technological advancements are extraordinary and have created a contemporary society that is remarkably efficient at supplying life comforts and entertainment, but the gains are balanced against the more hidden costs: "While the principle of work for the sake of the accumulation of capital objectively is of enormous value for the progress of mankind, subjectively it has made man work for extrapersonal ends, made him a servant to the very machine he built, and thereby has given him a feeling of personal insignificance and powerlessness."[7]

2. In contrast to the optimism that democracy would proliferate following the fall of the Soviet Union, we are witnessing a startling global rise in authoritarian, nationalist, anti-immigrant movements paralleled only by the rise of Nazism that accompanied Fromm's writing *Escape from Freedom*. We will do well to apply Fromm's insights to the present day by understanding the rise in authoritarianism as a function of societal failures that has led to a recurrence of an escape from freedom. As Fromm cautioned, "there is no greater mistake and no graver danger than not to see that in our own society we are faced with the same phenomenon that is fertile soil for the rise of fascism anywhere: The insignificance and powerlessness of the individual."[7] Failure to heed this caution could unleash state-sponsored destructiveness on par with Nazi Germany.
3. Life is increasingly taking place in the digital realm, which is mediated by large technology companies with profit motives. Platforms such as Facebook, YouTube, and Instagram pressure consumers to subscribe to competitive, capitalistic jockeying for the most "friends" and the most "likes." Again, the result is mixed. Many millions of people love and feel empowered by these platforms and the democratizing ability for one person to instantaneously connect with many. To use Fromm's terminology, however, we might also do well to consider: What is the "distinctive libidinal structure" of our society? Fromm would likely emphasize the outsized role of marketing. We need look no further than the seamlessness with which people talk of their "personal brand" to consider how much marketing has penetrated our mode of being: "The character orientation which is rooted in the experience of oneself as a commodity and of one's value as exchange value I call the marketing orientation."[22] When people feel unable to psychologically develop, Fromm argues that they appeal to external barometers for narcissistic supply: "If the meaning

of life has become doubtful. If one's relations to others and to oneself do not offer security, then fame is one means to silence one's doubts."[7] Funk extends Fromm's caution by positing that marketing has *become* the meaning of life for many: "The orientation to marketing invariably means that it is not one's true self that counts—i.e., the true talents, qualities, needs, feelings, thoughts of a person—but rather what can be sold."[26] People want their life to seem good, which is sometimes valued over the subjective, private experience of feeling good. Technology feeding us information to passively consume threatens our ability to create original thoughts and therefore develop as psychologically full individuals: "We have radio, television, movies, a newspaper a day for everybody. But instead of giving us the best of past and present literature and music, these media of communication, supplemented by advertising, fill the minds of men with the cheapest trash, lacking in any sense of reality, with sadistic phantasies which a halfway cultured person would be embarrassed to entertain even once in a while."[28] Bombarded as we are with video clips, notifications, and news feeds, "we are constantly exposed to the noise of opinions and ideas hammering at us from everywhere," which is making it harder and harder for us to listen to ourselves since "in order to listen to the voice of our conscience, we must be able to listen to ourselves, and this is exactly what most people in our culture have difficulties in doing."[17]

There is an increasing awareness that our society is not working. Fromm helps us to explain why. But, unlike most cultural critics, he also offers some very useful signposts about what can help us to right the ship: "I believe his radical humanism can offer an important corrective to the excesses of the politics of difference, that is, to the emphasis on what divides us rather than unites us."[29] Fromm elegantly argues a similar point: "And I would say is that there is another way, namely. If instead of a nation, the human race were to become an object of narcissism: If people could begin to be proud of the human race, rather than to feel proud of part of the human race. And it is a very strange thing how few people, in spite of the United Nations and in spite of all the progress we have made, in many ways have a real experience of pride in the human race."[20]

CONCLUDING REMARKS

Fromm did not believe that people were good, but he believed that people had a bountiful capacity to be good. In a time when there is so much uncertainty, it is a helpful framing to remember that humans have agency to shape our destiny. The way things are, is not how they must be. Prevailing ways of being and living can and do change. In fact, at every point in human history, the world has become something different than what it was before. This is why historians say that the past is a foreign country. As Ortmeyer put it, "Hope, a close ally of faith, was a potent force in his thinking as a motivational determinant in adult life, stimulating personal growth, altruism and his views of society."[2]

Instead of lamenting that the world is careening in the wrong direction, Fromm advised to look at our world with a critical distance and said: It was not always like this. What did we have before that we do not have now that can mitigate this? This can also help us understand emergent phenomena that do not blindly adhere to the past but help to understand the direction of culture. We do not have the luxury to hear what Fromm would say about the current state of our society, but we can make some reasonable inferences: (1) He would be skeptical of populist and nationalist movements, where individuals cede their freedom to irresponsible authoritarians who have little respect for personal freedoms; (2) he would be skeptical of "influencer" culture that molds personality and personal expression toward that which is "monetizable"; (3) he would be skeptical of big tech platforms that create algorithms to feed people information and sell them products, which creates a circular loop of empty, consumerist bursts of pleasure; (4) he would be skeptical that social media creates a groupthink that one's belonging is contingent on acceptance of prevailing cultural ideas; and (5) he would lament the continuation of a society driven by success and productivity and not on love, belonging, and connection.

Fromm's ideas have aged well and are remarkably applicable to the present. Nevertheless, he is not without detractors, and some of his ideas must be met with additional scrutiny. For example, Fromm seems to assert without much support that individual love relationships are a defense against love for mankind. This seems more likely to be Fromm's personal life philosophy (and a productive one!) but not a universal truth. Achieving unity with all humans is a laudable ideal, but perhaps like the understanding of human smallness vis-à-vis the cosmos: Helpful framing, but difficult to grasp hold of for longer than a few seconds at a time.

Finally, Fromm's recommendation that we try to seek out a definition of mental health that is divorced from individual circumstance is a fascinating, useful thought experiment, but not easily applied. We can perhaps approach this through rigorous comparison of various societal frameworks over the span of human history, but even still, how does one understand the "true" humanistic pursuits apart from culture when Fromm himself concedes that the social is woven into personality from the start?

One might also be partly skeptical of Fromm's valorizing the iconoclast. Indeed, there are many reasons to resist an authoritarian movement, say, but one might wonder if Fromm has swung too far in advocating that people step outside their time and place. For one has no choice but to live in the era he was born into, and adaptation to that mode of living will, as Fromm says, be decisive in terms of his subjective sense of well-being. How much can we reasonably ask people to incur personal hardship by taking a stand against the prevailing culture, knowing it can and frequently does cast out voices of dissent? On the other hand, Fromm might say it is precisely those dissenting voices who will save us from our worst impulses, as Fromm himself did. Despite their theoretical differences, Freud and Fromm had this in common. Indeed, in his book about Freud, Fromm writes, "One of his most extraordinary qualities, his courage... The courage which is involved here is of a special kind... The courage to trust reason requires risking isolation or aloneness, and this threat is to many even harder to bear than the threat of life."[30] The same could be said of Fromm.[31] It will be left to future Fromm scholars to advance his concepts of the "universal" humanistic values and use them as the basis for critique of the social character and a new orientation of evenly hovering attention between the present society and the one we may aspire to in the future.

REFERENCES

1. Mclaughlin N. Revision from the Margins: Fromm's Contributions to Psychoanalysis. Int Forum Psychoanal. 2001;9(3-4):241-7.
2. Ortmeyer DH. Revisiting Erich Fromm. Int Forum Psychoanal. 1998;7(1):25-33.
3. Friedman L. The lives of Erich Fromm: Love's prophet. New York: Columbia University Press; 2013.
4. Ingleby D. Introduction. In: Fromm E (Ed). The Sane Society. New York: Rinehart & Company; 2001.
5. Fromm E. The art of loving. New York: Harper & Row; 1956.
6. Silver CB. Erich Fromm and the Making and Unmaking of the Sociocultural. Psychoanal Rev. 2017;104:389-414.
7. Fromm E. Escape from freedom. New York: Farrar & Rinehart; 1941.
8. Freud S. (1915b). Instincts and Their Vicissitudes. Collected Papers, IV. London: Hogarth Press; 1925.
9. Cortina M. Rethinking Erich Fromm's Humanism and His View of Human Nature. Psychoanal Inq. 2024;44(1):95-102.
10. Fromm E. Beyond the Chains of Illusion: My Encounter with Marx and Freud. New York: Simon & Schuster; 1985. p. 182, xvii.
11. Fromm E. Interview with Mike Wallace. First published in: Survival and Freedom. New York: The Fund for the Republic. No. 5; 1958.
12. Fromm E. Love in America. In: H. Smith (Ed). Creativity and Its Cultivation. New York: Harper & Row; 1959d. pp. 123-31.
13. Freud S. A special type of choice of object made by men. S.E. 1910;11:165-75.
14. Fromm. Psychoanalysis and Sociology. First published under the title "sychoanalyse und Soziologie," in: Zeitschrift für Psychoanalytische Pädagogik, Wien (Internationaler Psychoanalytischer Verlag). 1929;3:268-70. Translation into English first published in: Bronner SE, Kellner DM (Eds), Critical Theory and Society. A Reader. New York and London: Routledge; 1989. pp. 37-9.
15. Freud S. Civilization and its discontents. SE. 1930;21:1-273.
16. Freud S. "Group Psychology and the Analysis of the Ego," The Standard Edition of the Complete Works of Sigmund Freud, Vol. 18. London: The Hogart Press; 1921. pp. 67-143.

17. Fromm E. Man for himself: An inquiry into the psychology of ethics. New York: Rinehart & Winston; 1947.
18. Fromm E. Marx's concept of man. New York: Frederick Ungar Publishing; 1961.
19. Funk R. Erich Fromm's Legacy. Funk R, McLaughlin N (Eds). Towards a Human Science. The Relevance of Erich Fromm for Today. Giessen: Psychosozial-Verlag; 2015. pp. 99-110.
20. Fromm E. The Concept of Mental Health. Lecture. In: E. Fromm. The Pathology of Normalcy: Contributions to a Science of Man, edited and with a Foreword by Rainer Funk. New York: American Mental Health Foundation; 1962. pp. 81-99.
21. Buechler S. Erich Fromm: Clinical Mountain Guide. Psychoanal Inq. 2024;44:103-15.
22. Funk R. Productivity in face of a 'pathology of normalcy': Erich Fromm's contribution to Critical Psychology. Psychology of Everyday Activity. 2023;16(1): 31-8.
23. Freud S. Beyond the Pleasure Principle. SE. 1920g;18:7-64.
24. Frie R. Long Shadows of Racism and Genocide: Learning from Erich Fromm's Social Psychoanalysis. Psychoanal Inq. 2024;44(1):15-25.
25. Cortina M. Prologue: Erich Fromm's Relevance for Our Troubled World. Psychoanal Inq. 2024;44(1):1-8.
26. Funk R. The Continuing Relevance of Erich Fromm. 2000.
27. Fromm. E. Why is America Violent? First published as a "special to the National Catholic Reporter." National Catholic Reporter. 1968;4(33):1-3.
28. Fromm E. *The Sane Society*. New York: Holt, Rinehart and Winston; 1955.
29. Philipson I. The Last Public Psychoanalyst?: Why Fromm Matters in the 21st Century. Psychoanal Perspect. 2017;14(1):52-74.
30. Fromm E. Sigmund Freud's mission: An analysis of his personality and influence. New York: Harper & Brothers; 1959.
31. Erich Fromm. The Psychology of Normalcy: Dissent, New York, Vol. 1 (Spring 1954), pp. 139-43.

CHAPTER 3 Erik Erikson

Sarah Varun Vas, Andres J Pumariega

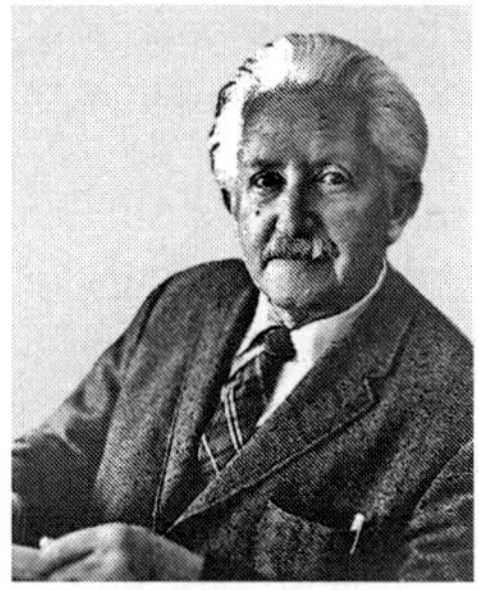

(1902–1994)

INTRODUCTION

In a life of uncertainty and unpredictability, at times we need just enough light to take the next bold step, the next sure foothold on a steep and rocky terrain. Yet, when the journey is complete, hindsight is the perfect vision, enlightening the understanding of why that arduous road, traversed with great care, had all those unexpected twists and turns: To end better than in the beginning.[1]

Erik Homburger Erikson, renowned for his theory on psychosocial development, is acknowledged as a pioneer in the fields of psychoanalysis and child development and merits this recognition in social psychiatry and cultural psychiatry.[2] Erikson's observations and keen reflections during his lifelong grappling with his identity and a need for belonging have deepened our understanding of the complex interplay of family, culture, and society in the development of identity and of purpose.[3] Contrary to Freudian teachings that personality is fixed in early childhood by the interplay of the identity, ego, and superego, Erikson's theories highlighted that the many facets of identity are formed by factors "outside of himself" (extra se), with the potential for growth and development throughout life.[3,4]

In this chapter, we will briefly examine Erikson's life trajectory and how Erikson's contributions are strongly influenced by the various people and groups he encountered and closely observed and learned from.[3]

TABLE 1: Notable publications.

- "Childhood and Society" (1950, 1963)
- "Young Man Luther" (1958)
- "Identity and the Life Cycle" (1959, 1980)
- "Insight and Responsibility" (1964)
- "Identity: Youth and Crisis" (1968)
- "Gandhi's Truth" (1969)
- "Autobiographic Notes on the Identity Crisis" (1970)
- "Dimensions of a New Identity" (1974)
- "Life History and the Historical Moment" (1975)
- "Toys and Reasons" (1977)
- "The Life Cycle Completed" (1982, 1998)
- "Vital Involvement in Old Age" (with Joan M. Erikson and Helen Q. Kivnick) (1986)
- "A Way of Looking at Things: Selected Papers from 1930 to 1980" (edited by Stephen Schlein, PhD) (1987)

We will ponder Erikson's pursuit of his own identity and the unique journey that gave him insights on his theory on psychosocial development, with its time-tested relevance in child and adolescent psychiatry, social psychiatry, and beyond **(Table 1)**.[1,5]

BRIEF BIOGRAPHY

Erik Homburger Erikson, named Erik Salomonsen at his birth on June 15, 1902, was born in Frankfurt, Germany, to his Jewish mother, Karla Abrahamsen, who learned of her pregnancy while vacationing in Germany. Escaping scandal, she did not return to her Danish hometown of Copenhagen; instead, under the care of her spinster aunts, she remained in Germany to give birth to her extramaritally conceived child.[3] Details about Erikson's biological father are still a mystery, and Karla held the key to that mystery safe in her own heart. Erikson's surname at birth was not that of his biological father; rather, it was that of his mother's estranged husband of 3 years, Valdemar Isidor Salomonsen, a Jewish stockbroker. About 4 months after Erikson's birth, Karla received the news that she had been widowed. She raised Erik as a single mother and studied to become a nurse. In 1908, she married Theodor Homburger, a Jewish pediatrician, who adopted Erik in 1911, an unexpected turn of events and the first hint of deception for the child who believed Theodor Homburger to be his biological father. Upon learning of his adoption by Theodor Homburger in 1911, Erikson questioned Karla, who explained that she was widowed, and he had been fatherless since Valdemar Salomonsen passed away in October 1902. According to his biography, even after his mother's death in 1960, Erikson continued the search for his biological father and discovered that he was an artistic, non-Jewish Dane.[3] Years later, Erikson still mentioned his mother's deception regarding the identity of his biological father, a foreshadowing of his own well-intended, yet deceptive attempts at protection. In Erikson's own words:

> *I grew up in Karlsruhe in Baden as the son of a pediatrician, Dr. Theodor Homburger, and his wife Karla, née Abrahamsen, a native of Copenhagen, Denmark. All through my earlier childhood they kept secret from me the fact that my mother had been married previously and that I was the son of a Dane who had abandoned her before my birth.*[6]

Erikson spent his childhood in Germany, where he was a fatherless child during his preschool years, a stepson during his early childhood, and an adopted son during middle school years. In his family, being the adopted stepson, his physical features contrasted with his dark-haired mother. In the community, his divergent appearance stood out within the monocultures prevalent in Germany.[3] His Jewish mother of Danish origin sent him to the synagogue, where he was recognized as being a Dane, with blonde hair and blue eyes; while at school, he was ridiculed for his Jewish heritage.

After completing his primary education, Erikson's adoptive father, Dr. Homburger, wanted Erikson to pursue medicine. However, Erikson's goals did not align with those of his father. Instead, Erikson, in his own words, reports that he *"indulged in what was then a German cultural ritualization, namely Wanderschaft, a more or less artistic and reflective wandering in which one sought some encounters with the cultures of the European South – and with great German writers (such as Freud...)"*.[7] He initially chose to study art for a year at the Baden State School of Art in Karlsruhe, Germany, where he also worked as an art instructor and tutor. He continued his studies for 2 years at the Academy of Art in Munich.

In 1927 in Vienna, Erikson's high school friend, Peter Blos, a budding psychoanalyst, was the director of Hietzing Schule, a private psychoanalytic school founded by Dorothy Burlingham and Eva Rosenfeld. Blos called on Erikson to move to Vienna and work as an art instructor and tutor at Hietzing Schule, under the guidance of Anna Freud, daughter of Sigmund Freud.[8] In Vienna, Erikson underwent psychoanalysis with Anna Freud, who mentored Erikson, discovered his sensitivity to children, and encouraged him to train in psychoanalysis.

In 1928, Erikson attended a masked ball where he met his wife-to-be, Joan Mowat Serson (1903–1997), a Canadian dancer and artist, who traveled to Vienna to complete her dance dissertation, which she abandoned to work with Erikson in Hietzing Schule. In 1930, the two were wed, Erikson became a husband, and just a year later, at the birth of his firstborn son, Kai Theodor Homburger, Erikson became a father.[3]

During his years in Vienna, Erikson's conflicts within his developing professional identity were apparent in his returning to the University of Vienna to study art, history, and psychology and, for a time, enrolling in medical school. He instead obtained a certificate from the Montessori School, founded by Maria Montessori, an Italian physician who was passionate about teaching and child development.[3] The Montessori method taught Erikson to look for the unique abilities and affinities that each child has for learning while encouraging the child's development and active learning in a supportive environment. He also earned credentials as a lay analyst from the Vienna Psychoanalytic Institute, where he studied psychoanalysis under Anna Freud. The years of mentorship under Anna Freud laid the foundation for the formation of Erikson's professional identity.

In 1933, Joan gave birth to their second child, Jon Homburger.[3] That same year, the Nazis had gained power in Germany and burned books authored by "enemies of the state," including Freudian literature. Erikson was practicing psychoanalysis, and being of Jewish ancestry and having two young children, he moved out of Vienna to Copenhagen, Denmark, to be near family there. After being unable to attain work permits or Danish citizenship, at the urging of his wife, in 1933, the Erikson family emigrated to Boston, Massachusetts, United States of America.

Erikson was among the first known child psychoanalysts in the United States of America. He continued his studies as a graduate student in the Department of Psychology at Harvard University and worked at Massachusetts General Hospital, at the Judge Baker Guidance Center, and as a research associate at the Harvard Psychological Clinic.

In 1936, Erikson moved to Yale to work in the Institute of Human Relations, where cultural anthropology, child development, and psychoanalytic theory were emphasized. Erikson went on to work in the Departments of Psychiatry and Pediatrics at Yale Medical School (what was later the Yale Child Study Center). Erikson's work was influenced by anthropologists Margaret Mead and Gregory Bateson, her husband. Margaret Mead, a close friend of Erikson and a cultural anthropologist, studied differences in child development and maturation through adolescence in various cultures and how these practices can affect the way an individual experiences adolescence.

In 1938, Erikson left Yale to study the Oglala Sioux on the reservation at Pine Ridge, South Dakota, including their tradition and the dynamics at play in the close-knit community, especially observant of the interactions between Sioux children and their mothers.

Around the same time that Erikson was working with and studying the Native American communities, he had an opportunity to legally change his adoptive name, Erik Homburger. In Native American culture, names hold deep meaning, linking the individual with nature and toward desired attributes; a personalized description, unique to the individual, which connects them to their community and future. Around adolescence, the young person receives a new name to help motivate growth and to establish their value to society.[9]

In the 19th century, patronymic naming traditions were common, where the children and grandchildren would bear the father's name and carry on the names of their paternal ancestors. In Danish culture, names carry significant cultural importance to the point that Danish law continues to regulate how children are named.

In 1939, Erikson and his family became naturalized as American citizens when he legally changed his name to Erik Homburger Erikson.[3] His first name, Erik, is the presumed name of Erikson's biological father. In keeping his middle name Homburger, Erikson honored his adoptive father, Theodor Homburger, while maintaining the Scandinavian tradition of naming his firstborn, Kai Theodor Erikson, paternal grandfather. Following Nordic tradition, he created the surname Erikson, meaning "son of Erik." Erikson's name change intimated his lifelong yearning for the man he never met, his biological father. Like the missing jigsaw piece that would not allow him to complete the puzzle of his identity nor satisfy his innate need for belonging, he crafted the name, "son of Erik." According to his biography, Erikson's son, Kai, was glad to escape from being teased and called "hamburger, hamburger."[3] The rest of the family members were also supportive of and gladly accepted their new surname, Erikson, for indeed they were already sons of Erik [Erikson]. While continuing to strengthen his professional identity, the act of changing his name and his nationality shed public light on his chosen family identity and his chosen national identity.

In 1939, Erikson moved to California to work part-time as a professor of psychology at the University of California at Berkeley (UCB). Erikson joined Alfred Kroeber, a cultural anthropologist and professor at UCB, in studying the Yurok tribe, as well as Mead and Bateson. His time with the Yurok Indians in Northern California also enabled Erikson to observe firsthand how cultural factors and norms contribute to the development of the psyche.[9]

A painful and private time in Erikson's life was in 1944 when Erikson's fourth child, Neil, was born with Down syndrome, and the physicians recommended institutionalization.[3] Unable to consult with Joan, who was medicated during labor, Erikson sought a second opinion from his friend and colleague Margaret Mead, who supported the counsel for his newborn to be institutionalized. Erikson heeded, and everyone was notified that the child had died during childbirth. Erikson's fourth child, Neil, lived until 1967 and had no interaction with his family. Years later, Erikson's children learned that their brother had lived in an institution for over two decades. (This reflects the lengths that parents will take to protect their children, and possibly even themselves, from distress.)

In 1950, the Levering Act, enacted as California law, required employees to sign a loyalty oath. Refusing to sign, Erikson resigned from his position at the UCB. He published "Childhood and Society,"[10] where he provided insights from his work. He expounded on the Yurok tribe, a group of fishermen and acorn gatherers living along the Pacific coast.[9,11] The Yurok performed a supernatural fish dance to aid their salmon fishing. Having a localized existence, despite intravillage conflicts, a joint cynicism toward outsiders was evident within the tribe.

Erikson's psychoanalytic observation of Indian tribes expanded his understanding that the development of the psyche is directly influenced by both individual and societal and cultural experiences throughout life.[9] Erikson illuminated social relationships in development with the concepts of mutual recognition and mutual trustworthiness that can be applied to successful development at every stage.[10] (Just as a mother's affection gives the child comfort in stage 1).

In 1951, Erikson moved to Stockbridge, Massachusetts, where he worked until 1960 in the Austin Riggs Center, remaining on as a consultant until 1973. In 1960, Erikson joined the faculty of Harvard as a professor of human development, where he was given time to continue his research and scholarly work while teaching, writing, and traveling.[3]

Erikson's work reflected his own constant search for knowledge and truth.[3,12] In his writings and psychoanalytic biographies, Erikson shares his candid observations of the practices and beliefs of various individuals and groups, including Luther, Gandhi, the Native American tribes, and others.[4,9,10,12,13] Erikson analyzed the lives and histories of influential leaders whose actions mobilized the masses and led to long-standing behavioral and cultural changes. In 1958, Erikson published a book revealing his in-depth psychoanalysis of the life of Martin Luther,[4] whose personal struggles and inner conflicts reflected Luther's identity formation, as he challenged the practices of the Roman Catholic Church.[4,12,14]

Years later, Erikson traveled to India to study the life of Mohandas Karamchand Gandhi, and in 1970, Erikson was awarded the National Book Award and won the Pulitzer Prize for his book "Gandhi's Truth: On the Origins of Militant Nonviolence."[3,13] Mahatma Gandhi is called the "Father of the Nation" for his crucial, nonviolent role in securing India's independence from British rule, earning the respected title, "Mahatma," meaning "great-soul" in Sanskrit.

Nothing is or exists in reality except Truth

—Mahatma Gandhi[15]

Erikson was nationally recognized for his scholarly contributions when he was invited to present at the Jefferson Lecture in the Humanities in 1973.[16] This lecture series was established by the National Endowment for the Humanities in 1972 and is still considered the highest honor bestowed by the US Federal Government and recognizes intellectual achievement in the humanities. In 1973, Erikson presented a lecture series titled "Dimensions of a New Identity,"[16] comprised of two lectures given on subsequent nights. The first lecture, titled "The Founders: Jeffersonian Action and Faith," on the "psychohistory" of Thomas Jefferson, a Founding Father of the United States of America, one of the primary authors of the Declaration of Independence, and the third US President who served two terms from 1801 to 1809. Erikson's second lecture in the series, "The Inheritors: Modern Insight and Foresight," was on the ever-changing American identity with her social, cultural, and psychological dilemmas.

Erikson's passion for learning was evident in his wide range of colleagues, teachers, and mentors, incorporating what he learned from leaders in various fields to expound on his theory of psychosocial development. In studying the development of the psyche, he highlighted the complex interplay of family, culture, and society on human behavior and development and the need to assess and understand the socioeconomic, interpersonal, and cultural factors that contribute to mental illness.[3,6,9,17,18] Erikson utilized a holistic view of the individual and observed the way each person is immediately influenced and/or threatened by his immediate and extended environments in every facet of development, stating, "the identity crisis in individual life and contemporary crisis in historical development because the two help to define each other and are truly relative to each other."[5] He concluded that merely understanding and treating the innate or biological aspect of an individual is grossly insufficient.[4,9,11,13]

Erikson was accompanied by and greatly influenced by his wife, Joan, whom he called "die Schone" (meaning "the beauty" in German).[3] Joan was born on June 27, 1903, in Brockville, Ontario, as Sarah Lucretia Serson. Joan's name changes may demonstrate resolution of her own identity crises, when she changed her name from Sarah Lucretia Serson to Sally Mowat Serson, to Joan Mowat Homburger at her marriage and lastly to Joan Mowat Erikson at her naturalization.

Joan supported Erikson's budding career in psychoanalysis, edited all his books, and completed his writings even after his death in 1994.[1] Joan continued to develop a ninth stage of psychosocial development and proposed this stage to occur in the 80s and 90s, when a person begins to decline and regress from all that they have gained through life, with the need for continued hope.

Both Erikson and Joan started out in the arts, painting, and dancing, respectively. Joan's interest in beadwork and basketweaving was likely sparked by the Sioux and Yurok Tribes, who transfer significant meaning to every aspect of each activity from one generation to the next, working together for the good of the larger community.[9] Joan recognized the need for continued learning and self-expression through art; she wrote books about community activities to build coping skills and resilience to promote mental and physical well-being.

Throughout the years, Joan developed talents in writing, basketweaving, and beadmaking. She published her first book, "The Universal Bead," a telltale of how much she herself was influenced by the Sioux and Yurok tribes, who used beads as a status symbol, as ornaments, and as currency.[1,9] For a time, she served as the art director and wrote books on how activity within the community is vital to recovery from mental illness.

Erik Erikson passed away in 1994 and Joan Erikson in 1997, survived by their children, Kai, Jon, and Sue, and his three grandchildren. The Erikson children continue to serve their communities in their respective fields.

MAJOR CONTRIBUTIONS

Erikson's first exposure to psychoanalysis was under the mentorship of Anna Freud, daughter of Sigmund Freud, whose structural theories described the identity, ego, and superego and focused on the instinctual, body-oriented, and sexuality-based behaviors of young children.[5] While Freudian theories described the ego as being a servant of the identity, Erikson's theory of ego psychology suggests that the formation of the ego as a complex integration of the individual's perception of self, which is constantly influenced by society's perception of the individual, results in a merging of interpersonal and sociocultural negotiations, successes, and failures, making his theories unique in the field of psychoanalysis.[6] The Freudian concept of the superego accepts that the child has internalized parental rules and expectations and the need for resolution of the conflict posed by the opposing forces. Erikson builds on this concept, articulating its intricacies in a meaningful and relatable way, providing multiple examples that enable the reader to visualize them.[5] Most uniquely, contrary to Freud, Erikson's theory describes ongoing growth and development as possible throughout a person's lifetime, with potential to resolve past conflicts and shortcomings with adequate support.

Erikson introduced the eight stages of psychosocial development, postulating an epigenetic model of identity formation, which required resolution of one stage prior to being able to fully resolve the subsequent stage.[10] Erikson's theory portrayed life as a series of unfolding tasks that occur in stages, describing a potential crisis with competing conflicts, more specifically the tug of war between the individual's desires and the societal expectations. On successfully completing a stage, the individual acquires skills and capacities, which Erikson calls "basic virtues," that lay the groundwork for successful completion of the subsequent stage, leading to the development of a healthy psyche.[10] Unresolved conflict at any given stage prevents the individual from progressing to the next level and hinders appropriate development of the psyche.

Erikson, in his book "Childhood and Society,"[10] synthesized elements of clinical psychoanalysis and cultural anthropology to discuss how the development of the ego is interconnected with societal and individual factors, which he called the mode-zone technique. He describes Sam, a 3-year-old child, with episodes of "violent somatic disturbance" as evidence of pathology that needs to be understood and treated. He expounds on the relationship between the development of libido, ego, and society. Drawing from Montessori, Erikson provides insights from his work with the Sioux tribes, the value and role of childhood education, and cultural achievements on personality development.

Introducing the concept of early ego failure, Erikson describes the conflict between identity and role confusion, which occurs during a crucial time.[5] Erikson provides a word of warning regarding the risk of emotional immaturity that persists in adulthood when childhood dependence is prolonged.[1,19] (In some Western cultures, the adolescent period has been significantly prolonged, with young adults remaining at home under the care of their aging parents. These mature grandparents are often the primary caregivers not only for their adult children but also for their grandchildren.)

The formation of a stable sense of oneself and one's place in society is vital in context of the environmental factors that contribute to growth, self-awareness, and identity. Erikson explains the human's desire for play and imagination throughout life, expressed through toys as children and through living out aspirations for a successful life as adults.[1]

In "Childhood and Society," Erikson went further in his formulations at a national/societal level to examine the identities of three nations: America, Germany, and Russia. He studied the exploitation of a nation he described as seeking a secure identity in history.[10] (This leaves the reader to wonder if individuals, families, and societies that are struggling to find their identity can be led astray by unbalanced or narrow-minded ideologies.)

Erikson's Psychosocial Stages of Development[10]

Stage 1: Birth to 1 Year: Trust versus Mistrust

Every child is born with innate, basic needs, including food and affection. During infancy, when the child's needs are met consistently and sufficiently, the child develops an understanding of the world as being consistent, learns to trust others, and develops the virtue of *hope* that their future needs will continue to be met.[10] However, when the child's needs are left unmet, the child will develop a sense of mistrust and learn to fear an inconsistent world.

Stage 2: 1–3 Years: Autonomy versus Shame and Doubt

During toddler years, children begin exploring their environment and discovering their abilities, such as walking, picking toys, and potty training. When the child is encouraged to explore independently, the child will gain confidence to develop the virtue of having *willpower*.[10] However, if they are made to feel inadequate in their exploration, they could become excessively dependent and begin to exhibit shame about themselves and to doubt and feel inadequate in their abilities.

Stage 3: 3–6 Years: Initiative versus Guilt

During early childhood, children begin to explore interpersonal interactions and to play with others. They learn to take initiative as their curiosity increases, and they develop a sense of *purpose* and security in making decisions with others.[10] However, if children are excessively criticized during this phase of development, they feel a sense of guilt, hesitation, and inadequacy in comparison to their peers. The child could believe that they are a burden to others or unwanted. To promote a sense of purpose and initiative in the child, parents and caregivers can encourage children to make choices and to act on them, for example, to choose their clothes for the day or the book they will read at night.

Stage 4: 7–12 Years: Industry versus Inferiority

During school age years, children spend most of their time in school, and teachers play a vital role in their development. During this stage, the child demonstrates the ability to learn new skills, start and finish a project, and develop a sense of pride and *competence* to gain approval from parents, teachers, and authorities.[10] They begin to develop an understanding of societal expectations. When a child is unable to meet the expectations placed on him/her, or if restricted from demonstrating his achievements, the child feels inferior, incompetent, and unworthy of society's approval. Parents and teachers can build a sense of competence and industry by presenting the child with age-appropriate, doable tasks.

Stage 5: Adolescence: Identity versus Role Confusion

During teenage years, the adolescent transitions from childhood to adulthood, with rapid and concurrent development in multiple domains. They begin to strive toward being independent while developing their own identity, either aligning with or rejecting their family of origin or other significant adults (usually a combination). They are exploring themselves and the world around them while developing skills to be an adult, learning their roles and how they will fit into society. They develop a sense of *fidelity* with successful completion of this stage and an alignment with societal expectations and norms.[10] When an adolescent is confused about their role in society, they might become rebellious and go against the expectations placed on them. Parents and teachers can encourage adolescents to explore their interests, allowing for self-expression and helping adolescents understand their roles in society.

Stage 6: Young Adulthood: Intimacy versus Isolation (18–40)

During young adulthood, the journey is to build close, lasting relationships and to find *love* and intimacy in sharing oneself with others. Having a stable sense of identity is important to being successful in this stage.[10] When successful, the individual develops long-lasting bonds with others, in a safe and secure relationship. However, without a stable sense of identity, the individual will find it difficult to form close relationships and might cause the person to feel loneliness, isolation, and depression.

Stage 7: Adulthood: Generativity versus Stagnation (40–65)

During middle adulthood, family and community are central to life and related to the preservation and transmission of human goodness. During this stage, the adult demonstrates *care* for both their young children and their aging parents while also positively contributing to their communities and growing relationships within the community.[10] When pursuits during this stage are merely self-centered and performed in isolation, a sense of stagnation mounts, leading to a disconnect with society, with a guilty realization later in life.

Stage 8: Elders: Integrity versus Despair (65+)

During this stage, self-reflection occurs, and the individual observes his/her life to reflect on worthwhile accomplishments and to find evidence of attained *wisdom*.[10] When successful, the individual reflects on life with positivity and closure. She/he gains a sense of completeness, acceptance, satisfaction, and integrity. On the other hand, guilt, regret, and dissatisfaction plague the person who has failed to find himself and has failed to serve his family and his community in a meaningful way.

Stage 9: Despair and Integrity (80s and 90s)

This last stage was proposed by the Erikson couple during their 80s and 90s. In their book "The Life Cycle Completed (Extended version)," which Joan completed and published after Erikson's death,[1] it stated, "*Old age in one's eighties and nineties brings with it new demands, reevaluations, and daily difficulties. These concerns can only be adequately discussed, and confronted, by designating a new ninth stage to clarify the challenges.*" Mrs Erikson described a *decline* in bodily functions and a gradual loss of the gains made in all the preceding stages of development, including loss of autonomy, self-esteem, and confidence, though without losing hope.

In the first four stages of development, the child is primarily exposed to his primary culture, a protected environment, once limited to home, school, and community activities.[10] Parents and teachers play a key role in protecting their exposure to the dangers of society, providing security and structure. With the advancement of technology and with young children having early access to the internet, cultural inculcation is quickly dissipating.

As the individual progresses through the last four stages of psychosocial development, she/he becomes increasingly attuned to her/his roles within society and to societal expectations, with their inequalities and instabilities.[5] With the completion of each successive stage, the role and contributions of the individual progress by not only taking care of self, home, and work but also a growing sense of duty to give back to society.[16]

CURRENT RELEVANCE

Erikson is the first known psychoanalyst to theorize that development continues throughout all stages of life.[1,10,19] His stages of psychosocial development contribute to our understanding of human development and are taught in many fields, including education, psychology, sociology, pediatrics, and psychiatry. Understanding Erikson's theory is foundational to understanding child development and enables the clinical provider to identify conflicts during each developmental stage while teaching skills to help the individual successfully overcome challenges and progress to the next stage. With the completion of each successive stage, the role and contributions of the individual progress not only by taking care of self, home, and work but also by a growing sense of duty to contribute to society.[12]

Psychiatrists and psychologists are trained to conduct a thorough biopsychosocial assessment of all the contributing factors while also understanding family dynamics in the context of cultural and societal influences as crucial to accurate formulation and treatment planning of mental illness.[18,20-23] Erikson's developmental theory, with its educational, clinical, and practical implications, enables parents, educators, and healthcare providers to understand which conflicts need to be resolved at each stage of development.[10] Involving the family in treatment aids the physician in understanding their diverse needs and the areas of vulnerability and strengths that contribute to the patient's illness.[24] For example, a dysfunctional family dynamic contributes to mental illness in family members, while mental illness in even one family member can add stress to the family system. It is important to recommend treatment for the family, including psychoeducation to build support, communication, and joint decision-making to strengthen family bonds and to promote mental health.

In his own lifelong pursuit of identity, belonging, and purpose, Erikson brought to light some of the complex underpinnings of demands and influences of culture and society on the development of the human psyche.[5,10,17] This correlates with the identity versus role confusion stage, where adolescents learn to understand themselves, considering the societal roles outlined for them.

The term "identity" was first used by Victor Tausk, a Jewish psychoanalyst from Austria, who succumbed to his own internal struggles with his own untreated mental illness. when he took his own life at the age of 40.[25] News of Tausk's suicide attempt was devastating to the community and coincided with the year of his publication "Influencing Machine," a singular case study of a patient, Natalija, having mixed delusions with fixed false beliefs that a machine was controlling her. Tausk's writings explained the intrapersonal struggles and thoughts, many of which were hyperfocused on the self, based on projection of the person's negative thought distortions and their perceptual disturbances rather than on fact and potentially triggered by exposure to traumatic experiences.[26]

> *The evolution by distortion of the human apparatus into a machine is a projection that corresponds to the development of the pathological process which converts the ego into a diffuse sexual being or—into a genital, a machine independent of the aims of the ego and subordinated to a foreign will.*[25]

Years after Tausk's death, Erikson revived Tausk's concept of "identity" and expanded on it.[25] Tausk identified the "pathological process" of hyperfocusing merely on self, with an intense attention to personal sensations while battling in an intrapersonal struggle and demonstrating a lack of internal control. With the advancement of neuroscience and pathophysiology, we are now aware of the potential for reward pathways to be activated to an extent where the response to these pathways is no longer under the control of the person, rather automatically and pathologically exercised despite negative consequences, requiring treatment for recovery.[27] The answer to this is looking outside oneself, to appropriately contribute to society and to her expectations. Erikson held civic institutions of family, education, and career, publishing his findings throughout his search for knowledge and truth. Erikson recognized that independent and exterior forces contributed to the development of the psyche and identity.[4,6,9,13,17]

Erikson's friend since adolescence, Peter Blos,[8] trained as a psychoanalyst and wrote a book, "On Adolescence: A Psychoanalytic Interpretation" (1962). Blos collaborated with Erikson in studying adolescence, expanding Freudian ideas, and viewing adolescence as turbulent; Erikson's later writings elaborated on adolescence as a critical synthetic stage of development. In his book,[5] Erikson highlights the identity struggles that adolescents face to balance personal individuality and societal value and belonging and the importance of ethnic/cultural identity in achieving an integrated identity.[5]

> *No wonder that Indian children, forced to live by both those plans, often seem blocked in their expectations and paralyzed in their ambitions. For the growing child must derive a vitalizing sense of reality from the awareness that his individual way of mastering experience, his ego synthesis, is a successful variant of group identity and is in accord with its space-time and life plan.*[5]

Erikson's resilience and perseverance against all odds become evident, motivated by his lifelong pursuit of what it means to belong and his search for knowledge and truth.[4,13] His developing a sense of self, of purpose, and of connection to his own heritage helped navigate this stage.[6] Erikson discussed themes such as the epigenesis of identity, which develops starting in infancy to adolescence and throughout life. He also discussed cases of identity confusion and the cultural components that affect identity formation.[5] The concept of identity is a mental representation of the individual's past experiences, present situation, and future ambitions.[10] Erikson emphasizes that the formation of a stable identity is necessary for the development of healthy and resilient psychological functioning throughout life. Identity formation is crucial to normal development and incorporates individual, familial, cultural, and societal identities.[5] An individual's self-worth, values, and purpose in community need to be addressed and resolved, not only during adolescence but also during subsequent stages throughout life.[1] When a stable identity is not attained, identity crisis develops, with ensuing confusion and uncertainty, lacking the skills to make informed decisions about future goals. Erikson's references in "Childhood and Society"[10] posits a similar challenge for societies and nations in resolving their collective identity.

Culture plays a crucial role in the development of society as well as individual identity.[3,5,6,17] According to the Practice Parameter for Cultural Competence in Child and Adolescent Psychiatric Practice,[28] culture is defined as an "integrated pattern of human behaviors including thoughts, communication, actions, customs, beliefs, values, and institutions of a racial, ethnic, religious, or social nature." We all play roles within society, at home, at work, and within our communities.[9,11,29] The diverse cultures within a nation with exclusive traditions, attitudes, and behaviors follow unspoken rules that influence how a person will conduct themselves within that culture. The members of the group hold similar values and beliefs, which affect accepted behaviors. Individualistic cultures prioritize personal achievements and independence, while communal cultures build ties between individuals and collective support.[23] By aligning to social norms, an individual can gain a sense of purpose within society and cultural acceptance.

Developing a stable understanding and acceptance of oneself, i.e., one's identity as an individual, and to belong to and have a positive impression of one's broader community and culture, is crucial to psychological health.[5] Erikson's keen observation, with its almost prophetic foretelling, of the challenges faced by Native American youth brought to light the important role of cultural identity, especially in minority youth.[9] Negative views about one's identity and/or culture of origin can promote mental illness. Acculturation stress, the stress from being directly influenced by two different cultures, can sometimes lead to identity confusion and to the development of mental illness. Frantic parental efforts to pass down family traditions and beliefs could be misperceived and even rejected by the adolescent. A living example, most evident in our day, is the technological gap that is affecting the generations and socioeconomic strata. As the younger generation takes their own journey of moving through the arduous task of chiseling out their own identity, we cannot discount the value of preserving a meaningful connection to one's origins, with the end goal of developing a secure identity in each of its facets, the ability to have shared experiences without losing sight of the foundational truths.[10] It is of utmost importance for families to find the common ground of shared experiences, being resilient to the changing pulls of society and culture, while preserving what is foundational.[30] We learn from Erikson and from recent research of the critical impact of cultural identity on psychological health (which he greatly influenced) that we need to remain sensitive to and ever cognizant of the cultural, racial, ethnic, and socioeconomic disparities that affect every individual, with the goal of improving policies and practices that promote mental health.[2,17,21,23]

CONCLUDING REMARKS

The year 2024 marks 30 years since the death of Erik Homburger Erikson and over a century since the beginning of his career in psychoanalysis. As one of America's first child psychoanalysts, Erikson's theories reflected his own pursuit of identity, and he courageously shared what he learned with the world.[6] His life and work teach us that psychosocial development is a lifelong journey with detours that can deepen our understanding of the world and of ourselves.[1] Erikson was very much a product of his times and familial/cultural background, yet few in the field have transcended their experience and applied the lessons from his life journey, as well as his academic work, to benefit our knowledge about the impact of social forces on human development.[12] In this manner, we consider Erikson to be one of the luminaries of social psychiatry.

Erikson's work deviated from that of Sigmund and Anna Freud to include external factors, including familial, cultural, and societal influences, in the formation of the psyche, emphasizing that the individual psyche, by itself, is not enough.[10] His theories and many publications depicting his own pursuit of personal identity and the eight stages of psychosocial development provided insight on the psychopathology that could arise from unresolved stages of development. The greatest gift that Erikson bequests to us is the hope that with adequate support, any identity crisis is not forever; every individual has the potential to develop a stable ego identity, and the potential for continued healing and progress throughout life: To end so much better than in the beginning.[3]

For decades, we have continued to examine Erikson's life and work to better understand our own unique identity and purpose. Out of Erikson's childhood struggle and need for belonging blossomed a passionate pursuit for identity and self, constantly influenced by how his society was shaping him.[3] With his wife by his side, Erikson amassed a substantial trove of understanding that continues to enrich us for generations.[1,3,17] It cannot be understated that with the advancement of technology, both societal and cultural shifts and strains will continue to impact the way that every person develops his/her sense of hope, of purpose, of acceptance, and of identity. We remain ever grateful to Erik Erikson for his enthusiastic and lifelong pursuit of identity, which has increased our understanding and has provided us with deeper meaning of the complexities of the innate need for a sense of belonging, the secret ingredient in the recipe for healthy development.[5]

Every person will face his/her own crises, that is the great opportunity of hewing and polishing out for him/herself a unique identity by expanding his horizons and continuing to learn about his world.[5] Erikson showed us how chiseling his own identity, in all its faceted brilliance, and by reflecting his wide spectrum of understanding of how he secured his identity for himself, for his family, for his community, and for the entire world.[1,3,5,6,10]

May our society strive to nurture its generations by honoring its heritage, by strengthening its family and social structures to enable every individual to attain his/her full potential. May each person strive to value his/her own uniqueness, to cherish the identity of self in all its facets (biological, of the body; psychological, of the mind; and spiritual, of the soul), and to strive for connectedness and duty to family, to community, to nation, and to humanity, and at the end of this intriguing journey on life's road, to have a secure identity founded in hope.[10]

REFERENCES

1. Erikson EH, Erikson JM. The life cycle completed. ME Joan (Ed). New York: W.W. Norton; 1997.
2. Gogineni RR, Pumariega AJ, Kallivayalil R, Kastrup M, Roth EM. The WASP Textbook on Social Psychiatry: Historical, Developmental, Cultural, and Clinical Perspectives. New York: Oxford University Press; 2023.
3. Friedman LJ. Identity's architect: a biography of Erik H. Erikson. New York: Scribner; 1999.

4. Erikson EH. Young Man Luther: A Study in Psychoanalysis and History, 1st edition. New York: Norton; 1958.
5. Erikson EH. Identity: youth and crisis, 1st edition. New York: W.W. Norton; 1968.
6. Erikson EH. Autobiographic notes on the identity crisis. Daedalus. 1970;99(4):730-59.
7. Erikson EH. Childhood and society, 2nd edition. New York: Norton & Company; 1963.
8. Palombo J, Bendicsen HK, Koch BJ. Guide to psychoanalytic developmental theories, 1st edition. New York: Springer; 2009.
9. Erikson EH. Observations on the Yurok: childhood and world image. Berkeley: University of California Press; 1943.
10. Erikson EH. Childhood and society, 1st edition. New York: Norton; 1950.
11. Grotjahn E. "Observations on the Yurok: Childhood and World Image." Erik Homburger Erikson. Int J Psychoanal. 1945;35(10):257-302.
12. Erikson EH, Coles R. The Erik Erikson reader, 1st edition. New York: W.W. Norton; 2000.
13. Erikson EH. Gandhi's truth on the origins of militant nonviolence, 1st edition. New York: Norton; 1969.
14. Capps D. Erik H. Erikson's Psychoanalytic Portrait of Martin Luther. Pastor Psychol. 2015;64(3):345-68.
15. Gandhi M, Narayan S. Selected works of Mahatma Gandhi. Ahmedabad: Navajivan; 1968.
16. Erikson EH. Dimensions of a new identity, 1st edition. New York: Norton; 1974.
17. Syed M, Fish J. Revisiting Erik Erikson's Legacy on Culture, Race, and Ethnicity. Identity. 2018;18(4):274-83.
18. Josephson AM. Practice parameter for the assessment of the family. J Am Acad Child Adolesc Psychiatry. 2007;46(7):922-37.
19. Erikson EH. The life cycle completed, 1st edition. New York: Norton; 1982.
20. Josephson AM. Reinventing family therapy: teaching family intervention as a new treatment modality. Acad Psychiatry. 2008;32(5):405-13.
21. Pumariega AJ, Rothe E, Mian A, Carlisle L, Toppelberg C, Harris T, et al. Practice parameter for cultural competence in child and adolescent psychiatric practice. J Am Acad Child Adolesc Psychiatry. 2013;52(10):1101-15.
22. Sharma N, Sargent J. Overview of the evidence base for family interventions in child psychiatry. Child Adolesc Psychiatr Clin N Am. 2015;24(3):471-85.
23. Rothe EM, Pumariega AJ. Immigration, Cultural Identity, and Mental Health: Psycho-Social Implications of the Reshaping of America, 1st edition. United Kingdom: Oxford University Press; 2020.
24. Livesey CM, Rostain AL. Involving parents/family in treatment during the transition from late adolescence to young adulthood: rationale, strategies, ethics, and legal issues. Child Adolesc Psychiatr Clin N Am. 2017;26(2): 199-216.
25. Tausk V. On the origin of the "influencing machine" in schizophrenia. Psychoanal Q. 1933;2:519-56.
26. Tausk V. On the Origin of the "Influencing Machine" in Schizophrenia. Sexuality, War, and Schizophrenia, 1st edition. United Kingdom: Routledge; 1991. pp. 185-220.

27. Herron AJ, Brennan TK. The ASAM Essentials of Addiction Medicine, 3rd edition. Philadelphia: Lippincott Williams & Wilkins; 2020.
28. Pumariega AJ, Rothe E, Mian A, Carlisle L, Toppelberg C, Harris T, et al. Practice parameter for cultural competence in child and adolescent psychiatric practice. J Am Acad Child Adolesc Psychiatry. 2013;52(10):1101-15.
29. Mann MA. The formation and development of individual and ethnic identity: insights from psychiatry and psychoanalytic theory. Am J Psychoanal. 2006;66(3):211-24.
30. Saroca K, Sargent J. Understanding families as essential in psychiatric practice. Focus. 2022;20(2):204-9.

PART 2

Sociologists and Anthropologists

CHAPTER 4

Geza Roheim

Behdad Bozorgnia

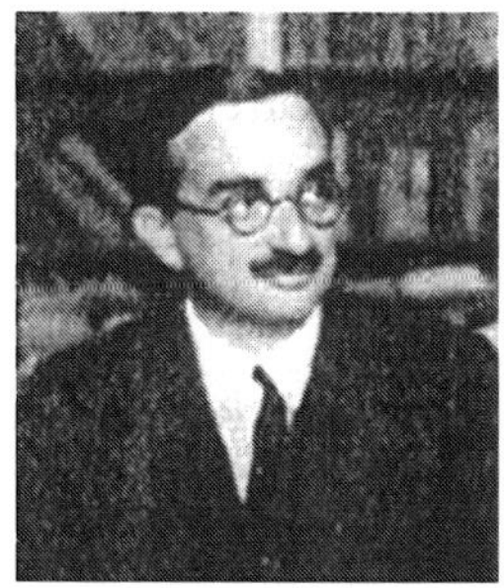

(1891–1953)

INTRODUCTION

Geza Roheim is not a household name and is less well-known in academia than some other scholars in this volume.[1] He is, however, a genuine pioneer in social science and psychoanalysis, being the first anthropologist and folklorist who had formal training in psychoanalysis. He took psychoanalysis outside of the consulting room and beyond the armchair to apply it directly to human behavior in the form of anthropological fieldwork. Although Freud often connected the origins of cultural and social phenomena to the unconscious in such works as *Totem and Taboo* (1913)[2] and *Civilization and Its Discontents* (1930), his work is often highly speculative or based on casual observation. Roheim took Freud's ideas about the unconscious determinants of human behavior and applied it to the ethnographic fieldwork of himself and others. He aimed to show that the unconscious was active in grand cultural productions such as art, literature, and religion and ordinary human interactions such as child rearing, medical care, farming, and trade. He further tried to see if psychoanalytic ideas were valid beyond the bounds of the Western culture within which they emerged by fieldwork with indigenous people of Australia, North America, and Melanesia. Although he is often recalled as a Freudian, emphasizing his reverence for Freud's ideas, his contributions have significant originality. If Freud is Copernicus, who watched the moon from afar and plotted its course, then Roheim is Neil Armstrong, who stepped on the moon's surface.

Roheim's understanding of human culture is boldly psychoanalytic to his supporters and rigidly dogmatic to his detractors.

BRIEF BIOGRAPHY

Geza Roheim was born in 1891 in Budapest, Hungary. He was the only child of prominent upper-middle-class Jewish parents who tended to overprotect and spoil him.[3] His father was described as stingy and trivial, while his mother was dominant and strong.[4] Although not part of the Hungarian aristocracy, the Roheim family's prominence and wealth cannot be understated. They owned their vineyard, and the family villa's first floor was rented out to Count István Tisza—Hungary's prime minister during World War I (WWI).[4] In a family interested in farming, business, and trade, young Roheim was severe and scholarly, preferring to exchange books instead of roughhouse with his childhood friends, among whom was Rene Spitz (1887–1974) who would later become an eminent psychoanalyst. As a young teen, his father opened a private account for him at one of the oldest bookstores in Budapest, where a clerk pointed him toward mythology and folklore. Portending his later career, Roheim delivered his first lecture about folklore to the Hungarian Ethnological Society when he was only 20 years old. Roheim was not a bookish academic but an accomplished athlete, winning multiple championships in table tennis, lawn tennis, and fencing.

While attending college at the University of Budapest, Roheim was drawn to anthropology; however, since there was no dedicated department in Hungary at the time, he pursued his interest abroad, in Leipzig and Berlin. He was greatly influenced by the 19th-century European Tradition of Anthropology, specifically the works of Edward Burnett Tylor (1832–1917) and James George Frazer (1854–1941). Both saw human nature as a constant and all cultures as undergoing a similar linear path of evolution. The universality and constancy of human nature underpin Roheim's research and contributions to anthropology throughout his career. During his studies, Roheim became interested in psychoanalysis as a way to understand the data gathered by anthropologists. He finished his doctorate in geography and anthropology in 1914 and joined the fledgling anthropology department at the Magyar Nemzeti Museum.[5] He began analysis with Sandor Ferenczi in 1916 and pursued his psychoanalytic training at the Budapest Institute of Psychoanalysis under his guidance. By 1919, Roheim became the first chair of the Department of Anthropology at the University of Budapest.

Roheim married a hospitable, charming, and funny Christian woman, Ilonka, in 1918. Roheim's family disapproved of the relationship, and the marriage resulted in a rift between Roheim and his mother.[4] The Roheims were an argumentative and querulous couple, often disagreeing and complaining about each other. They were, however, inseparable.[3] On one occasion, Roheim stumbled through a lecture to a group of candidates, which was not the norm. When his wife showed up, however, Roheim lectured smoothly. Ilonka was protective and contributed significantly to Roheim's career. She learned multiple indigenous languages, analyzed herself, and helped him in his fieldwork with women and children. When Geza and Ilonka were in polite company, they often spoke about private or contentious matters in either Aranda or Pitchentara, Australian languages they had both learned during Geza's fieldwork. They never had any children but remained married their entire lives.

During the first part of his career, Roheim was primarily an "armchair" anthropologist, applying psychoanalytic theory to folklore and anthropological fieldwork already gathered by others.[6] Although his application of psychoanalytic theory was unique, his conclusions were aligned with Freudian orthodoxy. In 1921, Roheim's paper on Australian Totemism won an award for significant research presented by Sigmund Freud.

Roheim would not formally conduct his fieldwork until 1928 when Princess Marie Bonapart, herself a psychoanalyst, sponsored him and his wife to Central Australia, the Normandy Islands, and the southwestern United States. In preparation, Roheim undertook a second analysis with Vilma Kovacks (Michael Balint's mother-in-law). He spent 3 years conducting ethnographic research with indigenous groups such as the Aranda and the Yuma, influenced by psychoanalytic theory and techniques such as interpreting dreams and children's play. The experience greatly influenced Roheim's theories of human nature and the genesis of culture. Although his scholarly career lasted much longer than his fieldwork, he drew on these experiences for all his future work. Upon his return from travels, Roheim finished his clinical training at the Budapest Institute, where he eventually became a therapeutic and training analyst.

In 1938, due to the encroachment of war and feeling threatened by the rise of both fascism and communism in Hungary, Roheim and his wife emigrated to the United States of America. He first settled in Worcester, Massachusetts, where he worked as a clinician at the local state hospital. He eventually moved to New York City, setting up a private practice while continuing his anthropological work and lecturing at the New York Psychoanalytic Society. Roheim's relationship to his country of origin was complicated. Although he never returned to Hungary and did not send any letters back to his parents, he described emigration as a "convulsion" and a "trying thing".[4]

Roheim remained quite prolific while in the United States, publishing many articles and books, including his most prominent works, *The Origins and Function of Culture* (1943) and *Psychoanalysis and Anthropology* (1950). He had numerous publications in *Psychoanalytic Quarterly* and *American Imago,* concurrent with very few articles in journals of academic anthropology. His ideas were marginal in the field of anthropology, however, they were

TABLE 1: Notable publications.

- Australian Totemism (1925)
- The Riddle of the Sphinx (1934)
- The Origin and Function of Culture (1943)
- Psychoanalysis and Anthropology (1950)

enthusiastically received and celebrated by the predominant branch of American psychoanalysis at the time. On his 60th birthday, Roheim was honored by the publication of a series of essays on psychoanalysis and culture, which included such eminent authors as Karl Menninger, Rene Spitz, Michael Balint, Heinz Hartman, Robert Waelder, and Joseph Campbell **(Table 1)**.[7]

Roheim only stopped writing when his wife died in 1951. Less than 2 months later, following a major surgery, he died himself. Reflecting their inseparability, Geza and Ilonka share the same gravestone in Woodlawn Cemetery in the Bronx, New York. The headstone reads at the top, "To My Dearly Beloved Wife" and at the bottom a quote from Horace in Latin "Exegi monumentum aere perennius regalique situ pyramidum altius" (I have erected a monument more lasting than bronze, loftier than the royal landmark of the pyramid)[8] since this chapter is about Geza Roheim's ideas and not bronze or the pyramids, he was perhaps correct.

MAJOR CONTRIBUTIONS

Geza Roheim's contributions to anthropology and psychoanalysis are twofold: (1) He articulated a developmental theory of human culture and (2) he expanded anthropological methodology to include formal psychoanalytic techniques such as free association, dream analysis, and transference. The content of his ideas about culture is as important as how he came up with them. In elaborating them, I will discuss Roheim's contributions to the psychoanalytic understanding of culture along the following topics: (i) The Ontogenetic Theory of Culture; (ii) The Boomerang of Progress; (iii) The Janus of Sublimation; and (iv) The Critique of Functionalism.

The Ontogenetic Theory of Culture

Roheim's initial ideas about culture are an extrapolation of the ideas in Freud's *Totem and Taboo* (1913).[2] In that essay, Freud contends that culture is a guilt-ridden reaction to primal crime whereby a band of sons murdered their father out of jealousy for his possession of the women in the tribe. The totem is a symbolic representation of the murdered father, and the bonds of society are a displacement of the original loving bond between the father and his sons. Freud presumed the primal crime to be an actual historical event and focused almost exclusively on cultural practices as a reaction to unconscious oedipal and triadic conflicts. Roheim's initial work on Australian totemism reflects the same manner of thought. In *Australian Totemism* (1925), he collected evidence in the form of indigenous Australian myths, folklore, and rituals to demonstrate the pervasiveness of father-son conflict in the unconscious. His initial work served mainly as an explanation and extrapolation of Freud's hypothesis.

Roheim, however, did not stop at being a mere footnote to Freud's cultural anthropology. Though he never explicitly disagreed with Freud's analysis, he eventually moved well beyond it. After his trip to Australia, where he was able to conduct actual fieldwork (as opposed to analyze the fieldwork of others, Rohiem expanded on the ideas of *Totem and Taboo* by (1) decoupling cultural practices from a particular historical event and locating them in an ongoing unconscious process and (2) adding on preoedipal childhood traumas and conflicts as essential unconscious determinants of cultural practices.

Roheim labeled his cultural theory as ontogenetic, denoting that the developmental experiences of each individual determine the meaning of cultural and social practices and vice versa. Childhood experiences (both in reality and fantasy) determine cultural practices later in life. Accordingly, culture determines child-rearing practices and, therefore, the fundamental experiences of childhood. The individual nature of cultures is based on paradigmatic experiences and traumas of childhood, which are particular to the pertinent culture.[9] Although Roheim's formulation regarding cultural differences is circular, his emphasis on the importance of childhood experiences in determining cultural practices is distinctive and fundamental. For Roheim, childhood was not a passing and insignificant phase of human development but essential to human nature and the cultural practices humans engage in. Cultures, whether in folklore, initiation rites, or agricultural practices, entail a series of compromise formations in response to childhood conflicts and traumas (both real and fantasized), i.e., the challenge of growing up.

Let us consider a few examples from Roheim's works. He offers an uncompromising psychoanalytic view of gardening.[10] He analyzes the practices of gardening by the Trobriand islanders, who plant yams by first holding and petting them while singing incantations about laying the yam in the ground like a mother with a child and having it grow like a suckling infant. Months later, the very same yams are dug up and split apart for further planting while they sing a different incantation about a husband hitting his wife, causing drops of blood to drop to the ground. The songs continue with the drops of blood gathering together and growing. In other incantations, the yams are referred to as blood, semen, tears, children, and excrement. For Roheim, gardening is not merely an economic practice necessitated by hunger but a ritual enactment of early childhood fantasies regarding destroying and repairing the mother's body, in addition to fantasies regarding parental sexual relations (the "primal scene"). Gardening is not just about having something to eat but also a chance for the return of childhood with its distinctive challenges and anxieties.

Importantly, Roheim applies ontogenetic analysis to indigenous and Western cultures. For example, he analyzes the modern idea and practices of nationalism or patriotism stemming from fundamental childhood experiences (1952). Patriotic songs and folklore use metaphors and symbols that demonstrate that the love of country connects to an idealized love and dependency on a desexualized mother. For example, Athena for Ancient Athenians and the Virgin Mary for early 20th-century Hungarians (and many other predominantly Christian countries) are conceived as maternal female protectors for the nation. In poetry and popular songs, they are paradoxically both maternal and yet virginal. However, this paradox is not problematic if viewed from the point of view of unconscious childhood conflicts where the mother is both an object of dependency and sexual excitement. For Roheim, patriotism is an elaboration of a child's idealized love toward their mother, which necessitates that the child's aggression toward her be repressed and the mother's sexuality be equally denied to avoid internal conflict and preserve an uncomplicated sense of dependency. The child's aggressive and sexual strivings toward the mother are generally displaced and projected (toward the oedipal father). In patriotism, these aggressive feelings are similarly displaced and projected onto a scapegoated outgroup, explaining the common trend from patriotism to jingoism and racism.

Childhood is fundamental to Roheim's understanding of human nature. He bases this assertion on the view that what is unique to the human species is the biologically determined experience of prolonged development from infancy to adulthood (Roheim, 1943).[11] The slowness of human development means that every human being must experience a protracted period of dependency on their parents/parent figures for survival, coupled with the development of sexual excitability well before both reproductive maturity (puberty) and the capacity for survival independent of the family unit. Therefore, each individual must contend with the inevitable conflicts imposed by object loss, which can result from reality-based trauma, i.e., anxiety from actual separation from the mother, or as a result of internal fantasy, i.e., aggressive fantasies toward the mother. Equally, as inevitable, each individual has to contend with infantile sexuality, which results in the internal conflict of the oedipal complex. All cultures (even matrilineal societies) develop in response to these fundamental psychic problems. The particular ways individuals navigate these conflicts determine the nature of their characters. Similarly, how whole groups navigate these issues determines the form of their cultures.

Roheim's interpretation of folklore from various cultures does not rely on a universal dictionary of human symbols. His idea differs from the universal symbology of Carl Jung (1875–1961). He notes that certain symbols are "potentially universal" but are not necessarily so. He argues that humans as symbol-making creatures who necessarily experience particular developmental conflicts often rely on a *potential* set of symbols to help them navigate the challenge of growing up. Therefore, some symbols are ubiquitous, but they are a matter of historical probability instead of inherent or essential meaning. For example, for Roheim, serpents in art and folklore are often phallic symbols, but this is due to an innate system of symbols or universally held set of symbolic archetypes but due to the universality of experiences of sexual conflicts and the ubiquity of exposure to snakes.[11] The association between a snake and a phallus is historical and contingent as opposed to inherent and essential.

Roheim's primary contention about the human condition leads to a vision of anthropology that is *radically psychoanalytic.* Since all humans possess an unconscious, psychoanalysis as a science of the unconscious is indispensable for studying the human species. The application of psychoanalytic theory and research methods represents a genuine innovation in the methodology of ethnography. Roheim applied such concepts and the pertinent techniques of free associations, transference, dream analysis, and the analysis of children's play to ethnographic fieldwork. Roheim *interprets* the rituals and practices of any culture as symbolic enactments of unconscious fantasies that are primarily related to repressed childhood experiences.[10] Roheim's ethnographic approach sees the content of his interlocutors' speech as free associations. He considers the relationships they develop with him in terms of transference phenomena. He further records and analyzes their dreams. All of this is to provide an account not simply of the manifest content of cultural practices but also explore the latent unconscious content behind them.[12] Notably, he engaged in a second analysis before his fieldwork, demonstrating an understanding of the importance of contending with countertransference in acquiring analytic knowledge. Roheim brought the analytic couch to the field, where it has stayed ever since.

The Boomerang of Progress

For Roheim, culture functions for society in the same fashion as neurosis functions for the individual: As a simultaneous defense against and gratification of unconscious childhood conflicts (1971). All cultural phenomena then, ranging from folklore to agriculture, can be understood as a response to the conflicts of growing up. As such, Roheim readily draws parallels between the symptoms and dreams of his neurotic patients and the folklore and rituals of particular indigenous cultures.

Consistent with many 19th-century evolutionary anthropologists, Roheim viewed the history of the species as directly paralleling the maturation of the individual. Accordingly, just as young children become mature adults, cultures develop from the more primitive to the more civilized. Therefore, the adult rituals and practices of primitive cultures can be studied as paradigmatic of earlier phases of individual development within a more civilized society.[9]

For Roheim, the more civilization advances, the longer individuals within that civilization stay children. The more civilized human beings become, the longer they remain infantile. Therefore, cultural progress by an entire society results in the delayed development of the individuals who comprise it. Thus, more advanced cultures require increasingly complex systems of defense to contend with the more protracted conflicts of childhood. He gives various examples supporting this, such as individuals within various primitive cultures reaching adulthood much earlier than their European or American counterparts. Although European culture is more technologically advanced than the Aranda of the Australian Outback, European individuals stay childlike for much longer. They are thus much more subject to regression in the form of neurosis.[9] The more an entire culture advances, the more individuals within that culture are prone to regression and neurosis. Cultures boomerang: The more they advance, the more they regress.

The Janus of Sublimation

Roheim's ontogenetic theory of culture leads to a unique and prescient perspective on the nature of sublimation. For Roheim, those who engage and create culture are engaging in the defense of sublimation. All cultures serve a psychic function in managing the conflicts of growing up. However, culture is not the only way human beings manage these conflicts. For example, neurotic symptoms also serve the same function. It is crucial to understand what separates those who develop neurosis from those who can engage in sublimation as a means to deal with their internal conflicts. To articulate this difference, Roheim describes the psychic substructure of effective sublimation and cultural practices.

For Roheim, cultural practices and artifacts work when they effectively serve as a midway point between ego and object libido, stabilizing the psyche in a prosocial manner. Cultural artifacts serve as substitutes for the love objects of childhood, therefore gratifying object-oriented libido and the need to quell separation anxiety. At the same time, since human beings make and engage in cultural artifacts, the process also serves to affirm and bolster the self. Therefore, gratifying narcissistic-oriented libido. Unlike neurosis, which gratifies conflicting drives and emotions at the cost of isolating the individual from the group, cultural practices allow for the expression of internal psychic conflict in a manner that affirms group cohesion (Roheim, 1943, p. 104).

For example, a person may develop a stutter as a compromise formation between her wish to shout at her father and her love for her father. The stutter turns the aggression impulse toward her father against herself and prevents her from yelling at her father, therefore gratifying her love for her father.

The symptom, however, isolates the patient from his family and society in general since others see him as suffering from a disorder. Cultural practices like sports, which often entail the competitive and aggressive confrontation of one group by another, also serve as another means to both gratify and defend against the awareness of the conflict-inducing aggressive feelings of childhood. However, the experience of watching sports brings whole groups together as opposed to setting the individual apart. The Janus function of cultural phenomena raises interesting questions about the ebb and flow of particular cultural practices as modes of sublimation with varying efficacy over time.

The Critique of Functionalism

Roheim's psychoanalytic view of culture differed significantly from the anthropology of his time. His basic assumption that human nature was universal and timeless, i.e., the psychic unity of mankind, was a predominantly 19th-century idea that was largely passed when Roheim published his work.[13] Roheim spends much of his work offering polemics of functionalism, specifically the works of Bronisław Kasper Malinowski (1884–1942). Functionalism explains each particular cultural phenomenon as fitting into a larger framework of institutions and practices that mutually support each other.[13] Therefore, a particular cultural phenomenon must be understood and analyzed exclusively in the context of its pertinent cultural framework. This naturally leads to a type of cultural relativism. Roheim criticizes this perspective not only for being superficial (insofar as it does not consider the unconscious) but also for making all cultures into isolated and self-contained units.

Interestingly, he posits such an approach is racist in its implications, simply replacing the idea of essentially different races of humanity with essentially different cultures. For Roheim, the unconscious is a unifying phenomenon for humanity. All human beings respond to the same impulses of the id but do so in various ways, which explains the differences between individuals and cultures. An approach that sees cultures as self-contained units is inaccurate and potentially unethical.

CURRENT STATUS

Roheim is relevant to both contemporary anthropologists and psychoanalysts. For contemporary anthropologists, Roheim's work with the Australian Aborigines still significantly contributes to that particular field of cultural study. Although Roheim's strict adherence to psychoanalytic orthodoxy still renders him unpopular in contemporary anthropology, his method of applying psychoanalytic ideas to studying human culture is steadfast in cultural anthropology.[14,15] Many contemporary anthropologists continue to use psychoanalytic theory and technique as an indispensable tool for conducting ethnographic fieldwork and understanding human nature.

Many of Roheim's assertions, precisely his assumption of the psychic unity of humanity, strict adherence to psychoanalytic orthodoxy, psychic reductionism, and Eurocentric point of view, have become passe in a world of postmodern pluralism and uncertainty.[16] Roheim's ontogenetic theory assumes that cultural evolution is linear, ranging from the "primitive" to the "civilized." His assumption that Western Culture is more adult while indigenous cultures are "primitive" and, therefore, childlike is patronizing and patriarchal at best and racist at worst. Such narratives, common in turn-of-the-century anthropology, have justified imperial and colonial projects against various indigenous groups.[17]

Yet despite these shortcomings, Roheim's theory has a complicated relationship to indigenous cultures. Firstly, his insistence on the "psychic unity of mankind" tends to undermine any argument for the supremacy of one culture over another. All cultures have various means of dealing with universal human conflicts. Secondly, although Roheim's framing of indigenous people as "primitive" is patronizing, he also was among the first Westerners to present how complex and nuanced indigenous subjectivity was.[17] Thirdly, his ontogenetic theory of culture specifies that as human societies become more advanced, the individuals that comprise them remain childlike for more extended periods. The regressive trends latent in cultural progress undermine any claims regarding cultural supremacy.

Indeed, according to Roheim, individuals in more advanced cultures are subject to longer and more intense periods of infantile anxiety (such as the threat of maternal loss, attack by a bad object, and punishment by the superego). Therefore, individuals in more "advanced cultures" are, in some ways, under more significant psychic pressure and are more prone to regressive trends on an individual and group level. Primitive people are healthier than their civilized counterparts. This claim, along with Roheim's emphasis on infantile sexuality as a determinant of human behavior, has led some to conclude that Roheim was a radical leftist, implicitly providing a basis for critiquing and changing the repressive and pathogenic tendencies of civilization.[6] Others disagree with radical leftist political inferences, emphasizing that Roheim's point of view was that of a strict psychoanalyst rather than a political theorist.[18]

Roheim's emphasis on the regressive trends latent in civilization's progress has fascinating implications for interpreting history. For Roheim, as civilizations advance, their members remain childlike for more extended periods of time and, therefore, more susceptible to psychotic mass movements, e.g., the rise of fascism and authoritarianism.[9] Although he never fully develops this idea, he lays the foundation for a cyclical view of human civilization whereby advancement creates the conditions of later regression.

Roheim's Janus theory of sublimation serves as a prelude to Donald Winnicott's idea of transitional objects, especially related to understanding culture. For Roheim, effective sublimation achieves a midway point between the ego and the object in a manner that stabilizes the relation among all parts. For Winnicott, transitional objects and phenomena delineate a space between the mind and reality and the self and others. It is a potential space where what is needed is both created and found.[19] Transitional objects allow children to individuate from their caretakers while developing an authentic sense of themselves. As individuals grow up, transitional objects dissolve throughout development, and their function becomes more diffuse. For adults, cultural practices serve as transitional spaces/objects between the mind and reality, between the self and others, allowing for authentic and creative living. Utilizing sociocultural practices as transitional spaces to achieve internal equilibrium is a marker of health.[20] Roheim's "Janus" theory of sublimation as a midway point between the ego and the object, which allows for stabilizing the self, parallels these later ideas and developments.

CONCLUDING REMARKS

Roheim was a pioneer in the field of anthropology and psychoanalysis. His extension and application of psychoanalytic ideas and techniques to the field of culture were unprecedented at his time. Although his particular eccentricities have rendered his ideas outside the mainstream of psychoanalytic and anthropological thinking, he remains relevant. As the burden of psychiatric illness grows globally and authoritarian political movements gather increasing traction in multiple societies in concurrence with unrivaled technological advancement, Roheim's ideas regarding the regressive trends latent in human progress seem more pertinent.[21,22] Multiple military conflicts and increasingly irreconcilable cultural and political differences plague our world. Even if his specific conclusions are no longer relevant, Roheim's vision of the unconscious as a unifying force across the incredible diversity of human ideas and practices still holds great promise and value.

REFERENCES

1. Spitz RA. Géza Róheim 1891-1953. Psychoanal Quart. 1953;22(3):324-7.
2. Strachey J, Freud A, Strachey A, Tyson A. The Standard Edition of the Complete Psychological Works of Sigmund Freud, Volume XIII: Totem and Taboo and Other Works (1913-1914). London: Hogarth Press; 1955. pp. 1-255.
3. Balint M. Géza Roheim. Int J Psycho-Anal. 1954;35:434.
4. Hárs GP. Géza Róheim: Alienness as a Source of Political Attitude. In: Borgos A, Gyimesi J, Erős F (Eds). Psychology and Politics: Intersections of Science and Ideology in the History of Psy-Sciences. New York: Central European University Press; 2019. p. 119.

5. Britannica. (2025). Géza Róheim. [online] Available from https://www.britannica.com/biography/Geza-Roheim [Last accessed February, 2025].
6. Robinson PA. The Freudian Left: Wilhelm Reich, Geza Roheim, Herbert Marcuse. New York: Harper & Row; 1969. pp. 89
7. Wilbur GB, Muensterberger W (Eds). Psychoanalysis and culture: Essays in honor of Géza Róheim. New York: International Universities Press; 1951.
8. Steinberg JJ. On finding Freud's anthropologists, Geza & Ilonka Roheim, in Woodlawn Cemetery, the Bronx NY. Bulletin of The Psychoanalytic Association of New York. 2021;59(1):4-7.
9. Roheim G. The evolution of culture. Int J Psycho-Anal. 1934;15:387.
10. Roheim G. The Origins and Function of Culture, 2nd edition. New York: Anchor Books; 1971.
11. Róheim G. The psychology of patriotism. Am Imago. 1950;7(1):3-19.
12. Róheim G. Technique of dream analysis and field work in anthropology. Psychoanal Quart. 1949;18(4):471-9.
13. Eriksen TH, Nielsen FS. A history of Anthropology. London: Pluto Press; 2013.
14. Groark KP. Freud among the Boasians: psychoanalytic influence and ambivalence in American anthropology. Curr Anthropol. 2019;60(4):559-88.
15. Hollan DW. Anthropology and Psychoanalysis: The Looping Effects of Persons and Social Worlds. Annu Rev Anthropol. 2022;51:155-71.
16. Elliott A, Spezzano C. Psychoanalysis at its limits: Navigating the postmodern turn. Psychoanal Quart. 1996;65(1):52-83.
17. Damousi J. Géza Róheim and the Australian Aborigine: Psychoanalytic anthropology during the interwar years. In: Anderson W, Jenson D, Keller RC (Eds). Unconscious dominions: Psychoanalysis, Colonial Trauma, and Global Sovereignties. Durham, USA: Duke University Press; 2011. pp. 75-95.
18. Calogeras RC. Gèza Róheim: Psychoanalytic anthropologist or radical Freudian? Am Imago. 1971;28(2):146-57.
19. Winnicott DW. Transitional objects and transitional phenomena. In: Winnicott DW, Masud M, Khan R (Eds). Collected papers: Through Paediatrics to Psycho-Analysis. New York; Basic Books; 1951.
20. Winnicott DW. Home is where we start from: Essays by a psychoanalyst. New York: WW Norton & Company; 1990.
21. Wu Y, Wang L, Tao M, Cao H, Yuan H, Ye M, et al. Changing trends in the global burden of mental disorders from 1990 to 2019 and predicted levels in 25 years. Epidemiol Psychiatr Sci. 2023;32:e63.
22. Doval GP, Souroujon G (Eds). Global Resurgence of the Right: Conceptual and Regional Perspectives. New York: Routledge; 2021.

Margaret Mead

Rachid Bennegadi, Rama Rao Gogineni

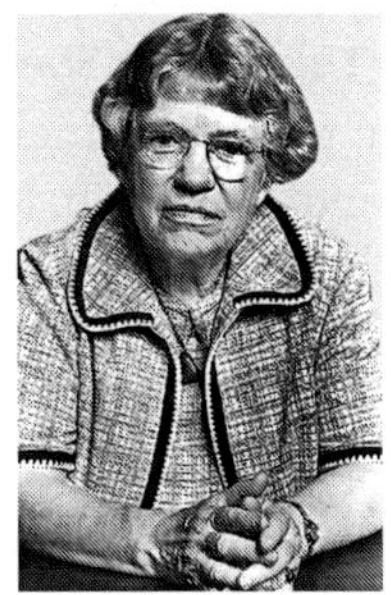

(1901–1978)

INTRODUCTION

Margaret Mead was an American anthropologist pioneered on topics such as childhood, adolescence, and gender and was a founding figure in culture and personality studies. Mead's contributions were significant and far-reaching. She conducted extensive fieldwork on various cultures, particularly in the Pacific Islands, and her studies had a profound impact on our understanding of human behavior and culture. She advanced fieldwork methods through the use of photographs, film, and psychological testing, as well as the use of teams of male and female researchers. She is best known for her studies of people of Oceania. She also commented on a wide array of societal issues, such as women's rights, nuclear proliferation, race relations, environmental pollution, and world hunger. Mead's work on Sex and Temperament in Three Primitive Societies became influential within the feminist movement since it claimed that females are dominant in the Tchambuli (now spelled Chambri) Lake region of the Sepik basin of Papua New Guinea (in the western Pacific) without causing any special problems.[1-4]

BRIEF BIOGRAPHY

Margaret Mead born December 16, 1901, Philadelphia, Pennsylvania, US—died November 15, 1978, New York, New York. Margaret Mead was the first of five children born to Edward Sherwood Mead, a professor of economics at the Wharton School of the University of Pennsylvania, and Emily Fogg, a former schoolteacher and sociology graduate student. Mead and her siblings were largely homeschooled by their paternal grandmother, who lived with the family. Mead had two sisters and a brother, Elizabeth, Priscilla, and Richard. Elizabeth Mead (1909–1983), an artist and teacher, married the cartoonist William Steig, and Priscilla Mead (1911–1959) married the author Leo Rosten. Mead's brother, Richard, was a professor. Mead was also the aunt of Jeremy Steig an American Jazz flutist. The Meads moved frequently to accommodate the parents' academic careers.[1,2]

Mead entered DePaul University in 1919 and transferred to Barnard College a year later. She graduated from Barnard in 1923 and then entered graduate school at Columbia University. She studied with and was greatly influenced by Franz Boas, the father of American anthropology, and Ruth Benedict, Boaz's student-turned-colleague. Mead received an MA in 1924 and a PhD in 1929. While still a graduate student, Mead began working at the American Museum of Natural History in New York City. During her time there she successively served as assistant curator (1926–1942), associate curator (1942–1964), curator of ethnology (1964–1969), and curator emerita (1969–1978). She taught at a number of colleges and universities, including Vassar College (1939–1940, 1940–1941), New York University (1940, 1965–1967), Wellesley College (1944), and Columbia University (1947–1951, 1952–1953, and 1954–1978), among others. She also served as president of the Society for Applied Anthropology (1949), the American Anthropological Association (1960), and the American Association for the Advancement of Science (1975).[1-3]

Mead's romantic entanglements were largely with other influential anthropologists. She married three times in her life. Her first husband, Luther Cressman (married 1923–1928) was an Episcopal priest-turned-archaeologist. Before departing for Samoa in 1925, Mead had a short affair with the linguist Edward Sapir, a close friend of her instructor. Second marriage is with Reo Fortune (married 1928–1935). Mead's third and longest-lasting marriage (1936–1950) was to the British anthropologist Gregory Bateson with whom she had a daughter, Mary Catherine Bateson, who would also become an anthropologist. She readily acknowledged that Bateson was the husband she loved the most. She was devastated when he left her and remained his loving friend ever afterward. She kept his photograph by her bedside wherever she traveled, including beside her hospital deathbed. Mead also maintained a close relationship, which some biographers have suggested was romantic, with her former teacher and fellow anthropologist Ruth Benedict until the latter's death in 1948.[2,3]

Mead's pediatrician was Benjamin Spock, whose subsequent writings on child rearing incorporated some of Mead's own practices and beliefs acquired from her ethnological field observations which she shared with him; in particular, breastfeeding on the baby's demand, rather than by a schedule.[2,3]

TABLE 1: Notable publications.

- Coming of Age in Samoa (1928)
- Growing Up in New Guinea (1930)
- Sex and Temperament in Three Primitive Societies (1935)
- And Keep Your Powder Dry (1942)
- Male and Female: A Study of the Sexes in a Changing World (1949)
- Blackberry Winter – My Earlier Years (1972)

Mead also had an exceptionally close relationship with Ruth Benedict, one of her instructors. In her memoir about her parents, *With a Daughter's Eye*, Mary Catherine Bateson strongly implies that the relationship between Benedict and Mead was partly sexual.[4,5]

Mead never openly identified herself as lesbian or bisexual. In her writings, she proposed that it is to be expected that an individual's sexual orientation may evolve throughout life. She spent her last years in a close personal and professional collaboration with the anthropologist Rhoda Metraux with whom she lived from 1955 until her death in 1978. Letters between the two published in 2006 with the permission of Mead's daughter clearly express a romantic relationship.[3-6]

MAJOR CONTRIBUTIONS

These references provide a comprehensive overview of the significant contributions made by Margaret Mead. Also mentioned are her collaborative works with Gregory Bateson to the fields of anthropology and systems theory. Social psychiatry was enriched by the extraordinary research done by Margaret Mead at a time where discrimination was affecting women, men, and children. Margaret Mead's Research Differed from Traditional Ethnology.[6,7]

Margaret Mead's research distinguished itself from traditional ethnology in several ways.

In methodology and fieldwork, Mead favored an immersive and intensive approach to fieldwork. She lived for extended periods with the communities she studied. During her famous research in Samoa, she spent several months living among the Samoans, allowing her to gather in-depth data on their cultural and social practices. Rather than conducting generalized comparisons across multiple cultures, Mead often focused on specific, detailed case studies. She placed much emphasis on psychological and social aspects, socialization processes, identity formation, and gender dynamics, emphasis on cultural influences on individual development, as seen in works like "Coming of Age in Samoa", and exploration of sexuality and adolescence from a cultural perspectives and role of gender in understanding of the cultural variability. Mead was an advocate of cultural relativism, a perspective that cultures should be understood on their own terms and not judged by the standards of another culture.[8,9]

She often integrated concepts from psychoanalysis and psychology into her analyses, highlighting the interactions between culture and individual personality. Mead wrote works accessible to the general public, helping to popularize cultural anthropology. Her work reached a wide audience and influenced popular perceptions of anthropology and non-Western cultures. Mead was also an active public figure, participating in social and political debates, and used her expertise to influence public policies and opinion on issues such as education, gender, and women's rights. In summary, Margaret Mead's research stood out from traditional ethnology through its immersive approach, focus on psychological and social processes, cultural relativism, accessibility, and impact.[10]

- *The influence of culture on personality:* Mead's work emphasized the significant role that culture plays in shaping human behavior and personality. She argued that many aspects of what we consider to be "human nature" are actually culturally specific, and that different societies can have vastly different expectations and norms for behavior. This challenged the prevailing view that human behavior is primarily determined by biological factors. She made use of work and observations from her fieldwork in Samoa where she embarked on a multifaceted research journey that encompassed the examination of America's national character. She sought to understand how culture influences and shapes personality traits. In 1935, Mead expanded her research horizon by authoring "Sex and Temperament in Three Primitive Societies," a comprehensive study based on her observations of the Arapesh, Mundugumor, and Tchambuli societies in New Guinea. This work compared the differences in sex roles, sexual dynamics, and philosophical perspectives across these diverse societies. Mead's research delved into the profound impact of culture on the formation of individual personalities, vividly showcasing the wide-ranging temperaments exhibited by men and women in different cultural contexts. For example, the Arapesh society was characterized by general peacefulness, while the Mundugumor society valued aggression in both genders. In contrast, the Tchambuli culture fostered submissive temperaments in males and assertive characteristics in females.[11]
- *Adolescence and cultural context:* In 1925, at the age of 23 years, she ventured to this Pacific Island, conducting extensive fieldwork. Her research culminated in the groundbreaking book, "Coming of Age in Samoa," published in 1928. Mead's study of adolescence in Samoa, "Coming of Age in Samoa," was a groundbreaking work that challenged the notion that adolescence is a universally stressful and rebellious period. She found that Samoan adolescents experienced a relatively smooth

transition to adulthood, suggesting that the challenges associated with adolescence in Western societies are largely culturally specific observed that Samoan children transitioned into the world of adulthood, including aspects of sexuality and work, with remarkable ease. This contrasted sharply with their counterparts in the United States, who bore the weight of Victorian-era restrictions on sexual conduct and an increasing separation from the productive world, needlessly complicating their transition from youth to adulthood. Mead's findings challenged prevailing notions about cultural determinism and the universality of human behavior. She argued that culture plays a significant role in shaping human development, marking a pivotal moment in the history of anthropology.[12]

- *Gender roles and cultural variation:* Mead's research on gender roles in different cultures helped to debunk the idea that gender is a fixed biological trait. She demonstrated that gender roles can vary widely across societies, and that they are largely learned through cultural socialization. This work was influential in challenging traditional gender stereotypes and advocating for gender equality. In addition to these significant works, Mead authored "Male and Female: A Study of the Sexes in a Changing World" (1949), "Anthropology: A Human Science" (1964), "Culture and Commitment" (1970), "Ruth Benedict" (1974; later edition in 2005), a biographical work about the anthropologist, and "Blackberry Winter" (1972; reissued in 1989), an autobiographical account of her formative years.

  Mead's exploration of these three societies collectively illuminated her conviction that variations in male and female personality types, both within the same society and across different societies, were primarily influenced by distinct cultural processes. These cultural dynamics varied from one cultural group to another or from one society to the next. In conclusion, Mead firmly asserted that culture's influence shapes the character, temperament, and personality of individuals within a group. Her ideas continue to shape modern discussions on nature versus nurture and the impact of culture on personality.[12,13]
- *Methodology and fieldwork:* Mead's fieldwork methods were innovative and influential. She used participant observation, interviews, and other techniques to gather data on the cultures she studied. Her approach helped to establish the standards for ethnographic research and has been widely adopted by anthropologists and sociologists.[14]
- *Public intellectualism:* Mead was a prolific writer and public speaker, and she used her platform to advocate for social justice and cultural understanding. She was a strong voice for women's rights, racial equality, and environmental protection. Her work helped to bridge the gap between academic research and public discourse, making her a highly influential figure in both the academic and popular spheres.[15]

- Then, Margaret Mead and Gregory Bateson were married from 1936–1950. Their collaboration was marked by an intellectual synergy that nourished their respective research, despite the personal challenges they may have encountered. Gregory Bateson's influence on Margaret Mead's work is evident through their joint fieldwork, the integration of visual methodologies, the contribution of theoretical perspectives on systems of communication and symbols, and their interdisciplinary approach. Their personal and professional relationship also contributed to enriching their respective contributions to anthropology. Their joint works resulted in "Naven: A Survey of the Problems Suggested by a Composite Picture of the Culture of a New Guinea Tribe Drawn from Three Points of View" (1936), "Steps to an Ecology of Mind" (1972), A collection of Bateson's essays on anthropology, psychology, and systems theory, exploring the interconnectedness of mind and nature, "Mind and Nature: A Necessary Unity" (1979) discussion of the relationship between mind and the natural world, advocating for a holistic understanding of systems and ecological thinking. Also yielded "Balinese Character: A Photographic Analysis" (1942), which combined visual and analytical approaches to explore the cultural and psychological aspects of Balinese society. Mead also learn incorporate, Systems of Communication and Symbols, socialization processes, and cultural transmission. Their joint work contributed to a better understanding of nonverbal communication, cybernetics and systems theory, human interactions and social dynamics, emphasizing interconnections and feedback within cultures. In summary, Gregory Bateson's influence on Margaret Mead's work is evident through their joint fieldwork, the integration of visual methodologies, the contribution of theoretical perspectives on systems of communication and symbols, and their interdisciplinary approach. Their personal and professional relationship also contributed to enriching their respective contributions to anthropology.[16]

CURRENT STATUS

- *Immigrants and refugees:* Mead's work enhances the ethics of brotherhood is to help someone with who we are and what we have by learning cultural codes and representations. Brotherhood is a surge without reserve, which transcends cultures, whereas solidarity in an intercultural context, is a surge to be completed by training, to achieve humanist objectives. To strengthen the patient/therapeutic relationship, we combine the notion of intercultural communication, intercultural mediation, cultural competence, and social elements training.[17-24]
- The ethics of brotherhood is to help someone with who we are and what we have. The ethics of solidarity requires one to go a step further, by

also learning cultural codes and representations. Brotherhood is a surge without reserve, which transcends cultures, whereas solidarity in an intercultural context, is a surge to be completed by training, to achieve humanist objectives. To strengthen the patient/therapeutic relationship, we combine the notion of intercultural communication, intercultural mediation, cultural competence and social elements training.[25]

- The clinical medical anthropology has a very particular aural context, and is a surge to be completed by training to achieve humanist objectives. Advantage in the understanding and management of the doctor-patient relationship in intercultural situations. When the caregiver or therapist has no control over the anthropological elements, this prevents him/her to indiscriminately dump his/her own nosographic and explicatory model that does not necessarily integrate all the cultural aspects. For A Kleinman (1993), it includes all changes and consequent physical and psychological reorganizations constitutive of the disease state. It is not just the patient's sole subjectivity as nonpatients increasingly share this as well. Therefore, it appears as a secular concept of the notion of the disease itself, its causes, consequences of his/her experience, and the means to address them.[26,27]
- With globalization and increasing migration, communities everywhere are increasingly diversified and aim should be to ensure diversity and cultural competence in all aspects of mental health care, but also to emphasize that mental health is as important as physical health in the policy of social development and the long-term integration. This way mental health services can facilitate adaptation and social integration of immigrants and promote cultural capital associated with diversity (Kirmayer, 2011). Mead's work with tribal, national, gender work is vital in understanding and implementing this.[28-31]
- Creating a multilingual, multidisciplinary therapeutic team integrating their competences in a complex intervention (for mental health: Psychotherapists and psychiatrists, anthropologists, cultural mediators, social workers, and community and clinical psychologists; women health and family matters: General practice medical practitioners and pediatricians, breast specialists, gynecologists, cultural mediators, psychologists, social workers, nurses, and anthropologists). The multidisciplinary and professional team is able to receive users from different nationalities or communities that have specific linguistic, religious, and cultural characteristics through using their first or preferential language and with consideration for their cultural representations of healthcare, of the body, and of suffering. It is up to the professionals to answer to specific care-seeking concerns: Diagnostic and therapeutic view, mediation, collaboration with other teams (particularly in the perspective of joint therapies), raising awareness in the approach of

concerned populations. Favoring pluridisciplinarity can also be achieved by including social services which will ensure/assist with healthcare access. Train healthcare professionals and operators within the "cultural competence" framework, and cultural mediation in the context of health care (the training should also be extended, when possible, to community health workers).[32-35]

CONCLUDING REMARKS

Margaret Mead's life and work continue to inspire anthropologists, scholars, and those interested in the study of human behavior and culture. Her research challenged established norms and helped shape the field of anthropology as we know it today. Mead's enduring legacy serves as a powerful reminder of the importance of open-mindedness, cultural diversity, and the ongoing quest to understand the complexities of human behavior.

As well as Karen Honey, Margaret Mead restored dignity to female psychology and open the gate of a new vision of globalization. In 1979, Mead was posthumously awarded the Presidential Medal of Freedom, the United States highest civilian honor, for her academic and public work. Margaret Mead, a name synonymous with the field of anthropology, left an indelible mark on the study of culture and human behavior. Her pioneering work continues to influence our understanding of the world and remains a cornerstone in the realm of social sciences.

In this article, we delve into the life, work, and Margaret Mead's contributions to the field of anthropology. At the age of 72 years, she attained the presidency of the American Association for the Advancement of Science. In 1979, even after her passing, she was posthumously honored with the Presidential Medal of Freedom, the most prestigious civilian award in the United States. Mead's influence extends far beyond academia. Her insights have significantly impacted education, feminism, and the study of gender roles. Her emphasis on cultural relativism and her challenges to conventional wisdom have contributed to the development of a more inclusive and multicultural society.

Never doubt that a small group of thoughtful, committed people can change the world. Indeed, it is the only thing that ever has.

—Margaret Mead[36]

REFERENCES

1. Encyclopaedia Britannica (Eds). (2025). Margaret Mead. American anthropologist. [online] Available from https://www.britannica.com/biography/Margaret-Mead [Last accessed February, 2025].
2. Mead M. (1935). *Sex and temperament in three primitive societies*. William Morrow & Company.

3. Mead M. (2023). Margaret Mead's Early Life. [online] Available from https://www.history.com/topics/womens-history/margaret-mead [Last accessed February, 2025].
4. Mead M. World Treasures: Beginnings; Shaping Forces—Margaret Mead: Human Nature and Power of Culture. [online] Available from https://www.loc.gov/exhibits/mead/mead-shaping.html [Last accessed February, 2025].
5. Howard J. Margaret Mead: A Life. New York: Random House Publishing Group; 1989.
6. Cassar C. (2024). The Life and Legacy of Margaret Mead - Pioneering Anthropologist. [online] Available from https://anthropologyreview.org/influential-anthropologists/margaret-mead-anthropologist/ [Last accessed February, 2025].
7. Vineeta K. (2023). Margaret Mead's Contributions. [online] Available from https://www.anthromania.com/2023/10/13/margaret-meads-contributions/ [Last accessed February, 2025].
8. Shankman P. (2019). Margaret Mead. [online] Available from https://www.oxfordbibliographies.com/display/document/obo-9780199766567/obo-9780199766567-0014.xml [Last accessed February, 2025].
9. Gordan J (Ed). Margaret Mead: The Complete Bibliography, 1925–1975. Mouton: The Hague; 1976.
10. Wolfskill M, Francis P. (2001). Margaret Mead: Human Nature and the Power of Culture. [online] Available from https://www.loc.gov/loc/lcib/0111/mead.html [Last accessed February, 2025].
11. Sociopedia. Culture and Personality Approach. [online] Available from https://sociopedia.co/post/culture-and-personality-school [Last accessed February, 2025].
12. Mead M. Coming of Age in Samoa: A Psychological Study of Primitive Youth for Western Civilisation. New York: Mariner Books Classics; 2001.
13. Mead M. Male and Female: A Study of the Sexes in a Changing World, 1st edition. NY: William Morrow; 1949.
14. Library of Congress. (1925). Margaret Mead Papers and South Pacific Ethnographic Archives: Fieldwork, 1925-1978; American Samoa; 1925-1926, Mead field trip; Field data. [online] Available from https://www.loc.gov/collections/margaret-mead-papers-and-south-pacific-ethnographic-archives [Last accessed February, 2025].
15. Nancy Lutkehaus N. (2003). Margaret Mead's Legacy: Continuing Conversations: Mead as Public Intellectual. [online] Available from https://sfonline.barnard.edu/mead-as-public-intellectual/ [Last accessed February, 2025].
16. Jacknis I. (2020). Margaret Mead, Gregory Bateson, and Visual Anthropology. [online] Available from https://www.oxfordbibliographies.com/display/document/obo-9780199766567/obo-9780199766567-0250.xml [Last accessed February, 2025].
17. Bhugra D, Littlewood R (Eds). Colonialism and Psychiatry. New Delhi: Oxford University Press; 2001.
18. Bennegadi R. Anthropologie médicale clinique et santé mentale des migrants en France [Clinical medical anthropology and immigrant's mental health in France]. Med Trop (Mars). 1996;56(4 Pt 2):445-52.

19. Bennegadi R, Bourdillon F. La santé des travailleurs migrants en France: aspects médico-sociaux et anthropologiques. Eur J Int Migr. 1990;15:129-43.
20. World Health Organization. (2015). Mental Health and Psychosocial Support for Refugees, Asylum Seekers and Migrants on the Move in Europe. A multi-agency guidance note. [online] Available from https://www.who.int/publications/i/item/mental-health-and-psychosocial-support-for-refugees-asylum-seekers-andmigrants-on-the-move-in-europe [Last accessed February, 2025].
21. Berry JW. (1990). Psychology of acculturation. In: Berman JJ (Ed), Nebraska Symposium on Motivation, 1989: Cross-cultural perspectives. Current theory and research in motivation. Lincoln, NE, US: University of Nebraska Press; 1990. pp. 201-34.
22. European Union Agency for Fundamental Rights. (2011). Migrants in an irregular situation: access to healthcare in 10 European Union Member States. [online] Available from https://fra.europa.eu/en/publication/2012/migrants-irregular-situation-access-healthcare-10-european-union-member-states [Last accessed February, 2025].
23. Carta MG, Bernal M, Hardoy MC, Haro-Abad JM; Report on the Mental Health in Europe Working Group. Migration and mental health in Europe (the state of the mental health in Europe working group: appendix 1). Clin Pract Epidemiol Ment Health. 2005;1:13.
24. Sargent C, Larchanché S. The construction of "cultural difference" and its therapeutic significance in immigrant mental health services in France. Cult Med Psychiatry. 2009;33(1):2-20.
25. Kleinman A. What Really Matters: Living a Moral Life Amidst Uncertainty and Danger. New York: Oxford University Press; 2006.
26. Bennegadi R, Bourdin MJ, Paris C. Les apports de l'anthropologie médicale clinique dans la relation soignant-soigné en situation interculturelle. La revue du soignant en santé publique. 2009;34:14-6.
27. Inter-Agency Standing Committee (IASC). (2007). IASC Guidelines on Mental Health and Psychosocial Support in Emergency Settings, 2007. [online] Available from https://interagencystandingcommittee.org/iasc-task-force-mental-health-and-psychosocial-support-emergency-settings/iasc-guidelines-mental-health-and-psychosocial-support-emergency-settings-2007 [Last accessed February, 2025].
28. Sartorius N. Fighting for Mental Health. A Personal View. Cambridge: Cambridge University Press; 2002.
29. World Health Organization and Calouste Gulbenkian Foundation. Social determinants of mental health. Geneva: World Health Organization; 2014.
30. Bhui K, Ascoli M, Nuamh O. The place of race and racism in cultural competence: what can we learn from the English experience about the narratives of evidence and argument? Transcult Psychiatry. 2012;49(2):185-205.
31. Bhui KS, Owiti JA, Palinski A, Ascoli M, De Jongh B, Archer J, et al. A cultural consultation service in East London: experiences and outcomes from implementation of an innovative service. Int Rev Psychiatry. 2015;27(1):11-22.
32. Dominice-Dao M, Kirmayer LJ. Cultural consultation in medical settings. In: Kirmayer LJ, Guzder J, Rousseau C, (Eds). Cultural Consultation: Encountering the Other in Mental Health Care. New York: Springer SBM; 2013. pp. 315-33.

33. Fernando S. Multicultural mental health services: projects for minority ethnic communities in England. Transcult Psychiatry. 2005;42(3):420-36.
34. Kirmayer LJ. Embracing uncertainty as a path to competence: cultural safety, empathy, and alterity in clinical training. Cult Med Psychiatry. 2013;37(2):365-72.
35. Kleinman A. Patients and healers in the context of culture: An exploration of the borderland between anthropology, medicine and psychiatry. Berkeley: University of California Press; 1981.
36. In 1986 a newspaper in Akron, Ohio remarked that the quotation appeared in a film titled "Women—For America, For the World" which was directed by Vivienne Verdon-Roe; the film later won an Academy Award: [online]. Available from https://quoteinvestigator.com/2017/11/12/change-world/#f+17220+1+7 [Last accessed February, 2025].

CHAPTER 6

Emile Durkheim

April E Fallon, Rama Rao Gogineni

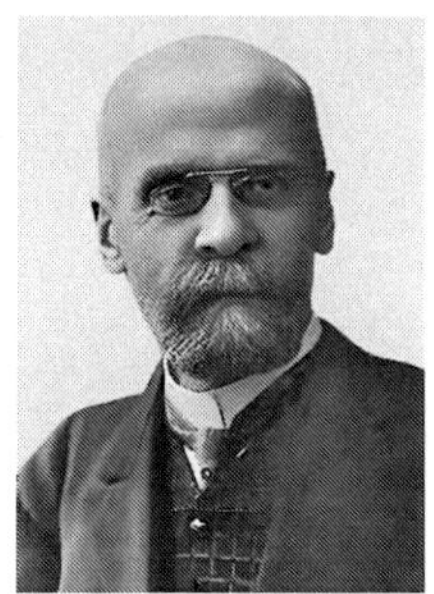

(1858-1917)

INTRODUCTION

As part of our understanding of human functioning, we acknowledge the importance of the larger sociocultural context into which we are born. This ineluctable initial framing of our world influences and spotlights our personal and professional queries and passions. Such was the beginning pursuits for David Emile Durkheim (1858-1917). Amidst tumultuous political, economic, and cultural shifts, anachronistic social structures scaffolded the transition to a new industrialized society; these elements fueled his interest in morality, religion, secular education, and social solidarity. He became later known as the Father of French Sociology marrying sociology with science. His theories and powerful positions influenced the next generation of teachers in France

TABLE 1: Notable publications.

- The Division of Labour in Society (1893)
- The Rules of Sociological Method (1895)
- Suicide: A Study in Sociology (1897)
- The Elementary Forms of the Religious Life: A Study in Religious Sociology (1915)
- Education and Sociology (1922)[11]
- Moral Education: A Study in the Theory and Application of the Sociology of Education (1925)[12]
- The Evolution of Educational Thought (1938)
- Sociology and Philosophy (1924)[14]
- Professional Ethics and Civic Morals (1950)

and left an indelible mark on the related fields of history, law, anthropology, and philosophy.

BRIEF BIOGRAPHY

Emile Durkheim was born into a close-knit, orthodox Jewish family of several generations of rabbis in Lorraine, France. Initially, he was destined to be a rabbi with his early years spent in a rabbinical school. With a German name and a Jewish heritage, he was subjected to an anti-Semitic atmosphere. This influenced his early thinking on the science of societies where Durkheim felt that this prejudice forced a tight bond with other members of the community which resulted in "each community [becoming] a compact and coherent society with a strong feeling of self-consciousness and unity".[10]

During his adolescence, Napoleon III declared war on Prussia, the Italians took Rome from the French, Russia broke a treaty and entered the Black Sea. Napoleon was defeated and captured by Germany. Lorraine was occupied by Prussian troops in 1870. A civil war in Paris ensued and was ruthless quashed by Bismark and hence the emergence of the Third French Republic 1871.[22] He was an exceptional student at the local college. After college, he left for Paris to enroll in the renown *Ecole Normale Superieure* to become a teacher. He was alone, worried about family finances because of his father's illness, and feared failure.[24] He became a somber and disciplined student.[31] After failing the entrance exam twice, he was admitted in 1879.

Durkheim was among a very elite and brilliant group of students. He became active in political and philosophical discussions and was a staunch supporter of the Third Republic. He criticized the Ecole's emphasis on literary rather than scientific study. Durkheim gravitated toward three compatriots and scholars (Charles Renouvier, Emile Boutroux, and Numa Denis Fustel de Coulanges) who supported his belief that sociology should be a separate domain of study with its own content and principles of explanation. In 1882, he passed the examination required to teach at State secondary schools and began teaching philosophy. For his doctoral dissertation, he studied the relation between individual personality and social solidary. By 1886, he saw this problem belonging to the new science of sociology, which required revising the methodological foundations of Comte.[22]

In 1888, he married Louise Julia Dreyfus and had two children, Marie Bella (1888) and Andre-Armand (1892). Louise was well educated and supported and helped Emile with his work. She was said to be light hearted in contrast to his austere demeanor. It is reported that they had a happy marriage.[32]

His interest in the study of "social factors" and an award by the French Ministry of Public Education led him to Germany, which had superior secular education. He wrote two articles praising the German view of economic phenomena within a social context and Wundt's view of the scientific study of morality. Durkheim brought back to France this ideology of restructuring education to be secular, scientific, yet embracing French morality. He was appointed in 1887 as "Charge d'un Cours de Science Sociale et de Pedagogie" at Bordeaux (1887–1902). His appointment allowed for "sociology" to become part of the university system. There was blowback as Durkheim highlighted the value of sociology in lieu of the humanistic transitions of philosophy, history, and law. The established professors feared "sociological imperialism" as Durkheim held that "metaphysical antinomies could be resolved sociologically".[22]

At Bordeaux, he lectured on theory, history, and the practice of education. He was considered an outstanding lecturer. Every Saturday, he also lectured to the public on various social phenomena.[24] These coalesced into *The Division of Labor in Society* (1893) which excluded him from the esteemed Paris professorship. Durkheim's early approach examined social phenomenon through the lens of evolution, history, law, and custom as the best indices of social structure change (evolution). Durkheim's early discussion of *conscience collective reflects his* notion that shared ideas and beliefs are forms of social organization. This was later replaced by collective *representations* which were more complex, differentiated states of a society's consciousness. His next set of lectures eventually became *The Rules of Sociological Method* (1895) where Durkheim attempts to establish sociology as a separate, discrete, autonomous science.

At this time, there was a dramatic rise in suicides.[33] There was popular discourse in European society that suicide had become a moral disease, which could be contagious to some members of the population.[35] Durkheim viewed suicide as a mirror of social malaise and a threat to social order. Durkheim, looking for a variable to demonstrate his sociological scientific method, chose suicide as he felt it was a well-defined variable. The topic may have in part emerged from his dear friend Victor Hommay's suicide. Le *Suicide* was published in 1897.

Durkheim was disappointed in the professional response to the publishing of *Le Suicide* and was noted to be thrown into a "slight postpartum depression".[34] He received correspondence such as "Basically, it is not so distant from social psychology…whether his egoism, altruism, or anomie are more or less conscious, they are nonetheless psychological causes…".[35] At the time, the medical press was silent, even though suicide was of interest throughout the century.[34]

One of Durkheim's most significant accomplishments was the founding *of L'Annee sociologique* (1898–1913), the first social science journal in France. With the aid of young scholars, the yearly journal reviewed areas that may relate to sociology (e.g., economics, history of law, etc.) and original manuscripts. Authors were expected to follow the framework of his *Rules of Sociological Method* (1895). Although Durkheim considered himself a socialist of the genre Jaures, he stayed out of the political fray. The one exception was the Dreyfus Affair where an innocent Jew (Captain Dreyfus) was accused of treason.[24] This involvement is likely what excluded him from being elected to the Institut de France, despite his academic contributions.[34]

When a position at the Sorbonne was vacated Durkheim became "*charge d'Un Cours*" and 4 years later, professor and chair of the department renamed "Science of Education and Sociology". He was considered a very good administrator.[32] In Paris, Durkheim was a powerful, but controversial figure. "His science of morality offended philosophers, his science of religion offended Catholics, his appointment to the Sorbonne... offended those on the political right".[22] His lectures were compulsory for degrees in philosophy, history literature, and language and the only required course for secondary school teachers, and thus earned him criticism of seeking "a pernicious domination over the minds of the young".[24] During his time at the Sorbonne, Durkheim's intellectual interests were in the sociology of morality, religion, and knowledge.[22] His later works on morality, *Elementary Forms of the Religious Life* (1912), and *La Morale* (published posthumously) transformed some of his earlier positions.

When Germany invaded Belgium and Northern France in 1914, he wrote documents sent to neutral countries to undermine the German propaganda. Durkheim was in poor health. "As a native of Alsace-Lorraine and as a Jew with a German named, Durkheim suffered aspersions of disloyalty motivated by the most vulgar kind of anti-Semitism".[22] A proud father, his son, Andre, was blossoming as a scholar. The biggest devastation of his life was when Andre was killed after being sent to Bulgarian front late in 1915. He suffered from a stroke and seemed to recover, resuming work on *La Morale*, but died in 1917 at age of 59. A number of his works were published posthumously and later translated into English.

MAJOR CONTRIBUTIONS

At the time that he lived and worked, Durkheim made a number of innovative contributions in France. Many of his contributions have transcended time and continue to hold sway in the fielding of sociology, psychology, and suicidology. While his founding of the discipline of sociology is his most significant contribution to the social sciences, his work on suicide is perhaps the most relevant and well known in the mental health field. Thus, it will be discussed first.

Seminal Work on the Sociology of Suicide: A Contribution to the Causes of Mental Illness

Le Suicide: etude de sociologie (*Suicide: A Study in Sociology*, 1897) was an effort by Durkheim to provide an exemplar of the scientific method applied to social phenomena that he had previously laid out in *The Rules of Sociological Method* (1895). *Suicide: A Study in Sociology* was to become a benchmark for subsequent work in sociology methodology and in the sociology of suicide.[35] Durkheim aspired to anchor his new field of sociology to the sciences rather than the humanities and philosophy. He selected to study suicide because it initially seemed like a discrete and measurable behavior. Official statistics on suicide had been collected beginning in early 19th century. Much of the data, a sample of 25,500 suicide cases, had already been collected.[40]

His work on suicide and the book went unrecognized for almost a half a century after its publication, even though many European governments were alarmed at the rising rates of suicide. It was hardly cited in Sociology journals until the 1950s.[34] Today it is a classic, read in courses of sociology and social psychology. It is a landmark study in the field of sociology, psychiatry, and for the study of suicide.[36]

Durkheim was attempting to connect relationship between individuals and the moral order of their society.[37] Durkheim frames his empirical study of suicide within his theoretical construct of the *collective consciousness*, real forces outside the individual which influence individual behavior. As Besnard defines the phenomenon, it is "in collective or social life, the production of forces or powers not given the individual organism... (which have a) distinctive character of the social fact versus its elements (i.e., the individuals)".[34] These are "emergent, distinct properties that are not reducible to the individual and her perceptions or decision making".[30] Durkheim argues that there is a complex process in which individual states of consciousness act and react to produce a new collective or a *sui generis*. These internalized representations compel individuals preconsciously to conform to customs and moral practices. One can infer their existence when sanctions are placed on an individual who does not conform.

Suicide: A Study in Sociology was the first major work to consider the influence of sociocultural context, inherent in the collective, on psychiatric conditions and in particular suicide. That is, membership in a specific group influenced the vulnerability of people to suicide based on that group's integrative and regulative characteristics.[30] About the phenomenon of suicide, he stated, "we will first seek the social conditions responsible for them; [we will] then group these conditions in a number of separate classes by their resemblances and differences, and we shall be sure that a specific type of suicide will correspond to each of these classes".[10] Durkheim observed that suicide increased at those times (months, days, and hours) where social life is most active and diminished when collective activity declined.[22] While he recognized that there is a base rate of suicide in every society, and these might be related to individual factors, he was interested in the variations of suicide occurrence which he believed were the result of the intensity of social life.[22] His focus was on the states of the various social environments (religion, familial, political society, and occupational groups).

In examining religious affiliations statistically, he noted that Protestants had the highest suicide rate, followed by Catholics and lowest were Jews. Here, he developed two lines of thinking. First that Jews, to protect themselves against the hostilities of the larger European societies, formed a closed tight knit group which enables members to better survive the physical and psychological abuse of antisemitism. Here, he draws upon his own experience growing up in a small integrated community needing to collectively battle the anti-Semitic atmosphere of both the French and Prussians as one united front. In differentiating Protestants from Catholics, he posited that Protestantism encouraged free intellectual inquiry, had less of a dogmatic creed, and was less integrated than its Roman Catholic counterpart.[22]

Durkheim theorized that the collective ensconced in an integrated societal structure protects individuals from what Durkheim termed *egoist suicide* or suicides resulting from isolation and lack of collective belonging. Integration occurs because of the recurring and ongoing social relationships which are embedded in larger networks that form groups and communities. Durkheim concluded that highly integrated religious groups protect individuals from suicide. Religion protects man from suicide because it is a society that adheres to "the existence of a certain number of beliefs and practices common to all the faithful, traditional, and thus obligatory. The more numerous and stronger these collective states of mind are, the stronger the integration of the religious community, and also the greater its preservative value."[10]

Similarly, Durkheim found that marriage has a protective effect for men (only), but the larger family unit provides immunity for both partners. Protection from suicide increases with increased family size, which Durkheim posited was the result of a greater number and intensity of connections.

The third social group examined was "political societies." Here, he contrasted early stages of society development with a more developed society. He reported that suicide was rare in the early stages, but increased as a society matures or disintegrates.

Durkheim referred to this resulting in excessive individualism which increases *egoistic suicide*. He stated,

> "The bond that unites them with the common cause attaches them to life and...prevents their feeling personal troubles so deeply... *Social man necessarily presupposes a society which he expresses and serves. If this dissolves, if we can no longer feel it in existence and action about and above us, whatever is social in us is deprived of all objective foundation... Thus we are bereft of reasons for existence; for the only life to which we could cling no longer corresponds to anything actual; the only existence still based upon reality no longer meets our needs...*

So there is nothing more for our efforts to lay hold of, and we feel them lose themselves in emptiness".[10]

There is consistent empirical support for this hypothesis across time, space, and disciplinary boundaries.[30,37] Where seniors feel, they do not have a place in society have increased risk for elder suicide.[27] Durkheim's economic and sociological variables in determining suicides are most applicable for white males, but not for white females or nonwhite males.[37]

At the other extreme of social integration is undifferentiated individuation. In these societies or groups, the individual has little value and the sacrifice of life is imposed by the group. Durkheim (1897/1951) referred to this as *obligatory altruistic suicide*. Durkheim noted examples of suicide among "primitive peoples" such as women upon the death of their husbands and servants upon the death of their emperor. Although less frequent, examples in "civilized societies" are early Christian martyrs and French revolutionaries.[38]

In contemporary society, there are numerous examples of communities where social structure is dense—cults and high schools where there is an emergence of suicide clusters.[21] Smith (1984) provides a poignant example in his report of Iranian teenage boys recruited by local village clergy, indoctrinated, then bound together by ropes to prevent desertion and sent weaponless into battle against Iraq.[39] They used their bodies to detect mines across the fields and hurled themselves on barbed wire. They wore headbands with keys attached to admit them to heaven. Other than these dramatic examples, this form of suicide has received negligible theoretical or empirical attention.[30] Both altruistic and egoistic suicides have at their foundation the extremes of integration of a society or disconnection that individuals have with each other. *Egoistic suicide* increases when there is excessive individualism and *altruistic suicide* increases when a society does not allow individuation.

Durkheim posited that the second factor governing suicide was society's degree of regulation which is embodied in the acceptance of norms, laws, and beliefs. Suicide rates would be reduced to the degree which the group's rules and social norms were coherent and clear and consensually shared. When a crisis occurs, abrupt changes in the social environment regulative functions may deteriorate or disintegrate. Traditional sources of societal regulation are religion, government, and occupational groups.

Durkheim uses the term *Anomie* to capture the condition of social deregulation. Durkheim attributed the increased rate of suicide occurring during his lifetime to the rapid increase in industrialization. This destabilized the traditional occupational groups. Durkheim believed that occupational groups provided much regulatory influence, for the individual knew the norms of the group and his place in society.[8] Durkheim believed that changes in financial status positively or negatively could increase suicide, as one's place in society is no longer applicable. Losing a job or financial standing would increase the likelihood *of anomic suicide*. The increase in suicide in 1929 after the financial crash is another contemporary example of empirical support for anomic suicide.

Anomie can occur in domestic life, as the social institution of marriage involves social regulation. Durkheim found that changes in marital status such as death, divorce, and other separations increase the likelihood of suicide.[10] Of this he says, “For by forcing a man to attach himself forever to the same woman it assigns a strictly definite object to the need for love, and closes the horizon” (pg. 270). For men, marriage provides “a coefficient of preservation... it does her less service than it does man where it is he that profits more by it” (pg. 274-275). However, with regard to divorce, there was an increase in suicide for men, but not for women. Durkheim speculates that marriage “is supposed to have originated for the wife, to protect... Monogamy, especially, is often represented as a sacrifice made by man of his polygamous instincts, to raise and improve women’s condition...(yet) he benefits more by it... it is she who made a sacrifice” (pg. 275-276). This is a particularly interesting acknowledgment given that he has elsewhere indicated that women are less well developed.

Whereas too little regulation can increase suicide, Durkheim posited that the other extreme of too much regulation may result in what he terms *fatalistic suicide*. Here, too much regulation may result in a future of suffering with no hope for relief. Durkheim did not expound on this notion and relegated it to a mere footnote. In contemporary western society, this kind of suicide has been under debate with regard to those afflicted with painful, progressive, and deteriorating maladies. Suicide for the elderly may fall into this category, in that with the decline of physical and mental functioning, there is less stimulation from the social environment and there is no hope for a change in role expectations.[23] He also found no relation between the type of suicide and the way in which the act was committed.

Thus, Durkheim empirically demonstrates the variable suicide rates among various social groups to support his theory that “that the structure of suicide rates is a positive function of the structure of a group or class of people’s social relationships and that social relationships vary according to their level of integration and (moral) regulation”.[30] He concludes that suicide like homicide is manifestation of a collective society breakdown.[8]

Throughout time, societies have vacillated as to whether to lawfully prohibit suicide by stripping the rights to burial, rights of titles, etc., for who complete it. Most religious groups throughout time have regarded suicide as a sinful act. As a product of his time, Durkheim too saw suicide as immoral, but for nonreligious reasons. Suicide weakens society in that the bonds between individual members are diminished by the act. In suicide, the individual does not “subordinate him(self) to the general interests of human kind”.[10]

Durkheim posits a moral theory of society organized around a symbolically troubling feature of modern life at the time, a generally accepted agreement that moral controls were decreasing and this was linked to the rise of industrialization.[35,38] Durkheim offers a society solution to this problem. He suggests that collective public projects will create protective structural changes, more effectively than trying to treat the individual. Such projects allow individuals to have purpose.

A century later, critiques of this study abound. The first involves the definition of suicide. Durkheim's definition of suicide was any death "resulting directly or indirectly from a positive or negative act of the victim himself which he knows must produce this result".[10] This definition counts acts of self-sacrifice as suicide.[38] Durkheim would include a soldier killed in battle as suicide, but officials may not document it as such. Thus, Durkheim did not establish the parameters upon which officials made those decisions and he was dependent upon how officials may have socially constructed the category.[40] Second, Durkheim presumed that his statistical findings of the differential rates of suicide among groups revealed accurate differences. Durkheim may have been naïve in his understanding of factors that could distort his findings.[40] Third, at the turn of the 20th century, there were no computers or calculators that could perform statistical operations which resulted in only rudimentary statistics by today's standards.

Fourth, Ramp (2000) noted that Durkheim used poignant and evocative language such as "overwhelmed and disorganized widowers" and "loyal military officers." In Ramp's opinion, "the contrast between these evocative passages and the starkness of the statistical analysis accounts for much of the rhetorical power of Suicide" (p. 86). This is, in contrast to today's standards of scientific inquiry, requiring the use of nonjudgmental descriptions.

The Founding of Sociology as a Scientific Discipline

During Durkheim's early professional life, the academic discipline of Sociology was nonexistent. Philosophy and history reigned as important academic studies in French culture.[22] In contrast to Hobbes and Rousseau, prominent philosophers at the time, who argued that the individual was real and society was artificial, Durkheim argued "there is in every society a certain group of phenomena which may be differentiated from those studied by the other natural sciences."[9] In *Les Regles de la methode sociologique* (*The Rules of Sociological Method*) (1895), he posits that the study of "social facts" is a real, separate, and autonomous science. He argued, "...we have the actions, the thoughts and the beliefs which uniquely exist outside each individual's own consciousness, and so provide a worthy subject for the study of sociology. Not only are these types of conduct outside the thoughts of the individual person, but they have a certain coercive power. If I try to resist it, I notice this quite readily."[9] He declares that Sociology is the scientific study of the social facts that exist in the collective consciousness of a society.

Durkheim conceived of society as a *sui genre* reality, that is collection of representations that is not reducible to its composed parts. Social facts are created when individual consciences interact and create a synthetic reality that is new and greater than the sum of its parts.[22] *Social facts* as Durkheim attempts to define them begin to have an elastic quality in that they include customs, rules, and religious beliefs. The structural features of society are where social functions are consolidated over a long time. As Jones (1986) describes it, *social facts* are an elastic construct, "covering the range from the most clear delineated features of social structure (e.g., population size and distribution) to the most spontaneous currents of public opinion and enthusiasm".[22] They can be recognized in social structures or culturally transmitted values transmitted through the generations. The coercive nature of social facts on the person can be seen concretely as laws or moral and religious beliefs that oblige or restrain someone.

In claiming sociology as a separate discipline from psychology and biology, society was a reality (sui genres) independent of the individual mind and body. In *The Rules of Sociological Method,* he concretized a methodology of study that would align the discipline with the sciences rather than history and philosophy. He stipulated that the phenomenon of study must be social, observable, and objective (independent of all doctrines, avoidance of social judgment). He distinguished a "normal" social fact from a pathological one by ascertaining that normal was what was seen in most and pathological would be found only in a minority. In the *Division of Labor* (1895), he identified crime as a pathological social fact. Durkheim authorized an endorsement of the comparative method of inquiry. His examples were comparing society at different time periods or comparing two societies at the same time period.

Durkheim further established the independence and importance of the discipline by founding the first European department of sociology at the University of Bordeaux. Through his powerful positions within the University, Durkheim was able to entrench of the discipline of sociology by inserting the study of sociology into the curriculum of those students at the University who desired to be teachers. Prior to this, education required study of philosophy and history. In fact, his Sociology course was the only course required by all students. By doing so, he was able to influence minds of secondary school teachers and the educational curriculum for many generations to come. He along with Karl Marx and Max Weber is considered the founders of Modern Sociology.

His fourth contribution to the development of sociology as a discipline was the founding of the first French journal of sociology, *L'Année Sociologique* in 1898. The journal was published once a year and it included anthropology, empirical qualitative and quantitative sociology, and book reviews of books from other disciplines that may be related to sociology. During his time as editor, the editorial team was composed of 50 research reviewers, some of whom were his students. They became known as the "French School of Sociology." Durkheim was fluent in German, English, and Italian, in addition to French and was able to review academic papers in each of those languages.[34] The journal is still in existence today, published continuously except for 1912–1916, during the war. It was relaunched by Marcel Mauss, his nephew and a well-known sociologist in his own right in 1917. The first issue included a eulogy for colleagues who died in that interim period and an essay by Mauss.[19] Today, it continues to publish papers on empirical sociological knowledge and research on social science history as well as research that highlights the relationship between sociology and other social sciences (*https://www.cairn-int.info/journal-l-annee-sociologique.htm*).

Theoretical Contributions to Sociology

Durkheim wrote and studied as Europe was engaged in the process of urbanization. Ensconced in this ambiance, his writings reflected a concern with how society is held together and functions when industrialization has the potential to erode and even destroy social norms. *Anomie* was coined by Durkheim to capture the notion of "a revolve toward or withdrawal from the social controls of society".[39] To that end, he focused on the interrelationships among labor configurations, morality, religion, education, and on social solidarity.

Durkheim, in his push for the separate science of sociology, saw society as a unique and real collection of representations that cannot be reduced to those parts that compose it, *a sui generis*.[10] Similar to a chemical reaction, society is formed when individuals with their internal representations come together, interact, and fuse to create a new reality, greater than the sum of its parts. He coined the term collective conscience to represent this collective notion and agreement of customs, rules and laws, beliefs, and other structural features of society such as rituals and ceremonies. He later broadened this concept and referred to it as collective representations.

How do we understand formation and maintenance of culture and society? Durkheim proposed that society was organized around the network of bonds between individuals and their society, the intensity of the individuals' connection to those bonds and the attachments that individuals have to each other.[39] His initial efforts contrast two kinds of social solidarity—mechanical and organic.[8]

Mechanical solidarity, usually present in more traditional societies, has organized connections to others with a shared identity. Everyone shares the same set of tasks and beliefs. For example, an agrarian culture may resemble this kind of solidarity where they are likely to share the same set of values and ideas. Here, individualism is discouraged, and ties are the mutual economic and domestic tasks they share.

The development of an organic solidarity occurs when the "dynamic density" increases. By this, Durkheim meant an increased population density, the growth of towns, and an increase in the network and efficacy of communication. When this happens, there is likely to be an increased division of labor, where individuals become more specialized in their skills and work. Individuality grows in that people who are recognized and needed for their specific skills and society becomes more complex. Despite a growth in individuality, individuals are less self-sufficient in that specialization that requires interdependence. There develops a greater feeling of solidarity with those who have similar jobs.[8]

Durkheim noted that the character of the laws present in each of these societies varies. Repressive law, which characterizes a mechanical society, is likely to punish based upon the damage caused to the social order. Restitutive law, which typifies an organic society, focuses on the victim with an emphasis on personal rights. There are specialized social structures and jobs such as courts and lawyers. Durkheim noted that as people are finding new social groups with co-workers, a collective consciousness diminishes. A more centralized authority needs to regulate relations between groups. The law also needs to evolve to manage social relations and civil law rather than penal sanctions are instituted.[22]

Perhaps, one of Durkheim's most important contribution was positing why the divisions of labored groups and institutions within a society would cooperate with each other. If one subgroup fails, there is a possibility of impending collapse for all others. Each group within the society must collaborate to ensure survival.[39] Specialized skills limit self-sufficiency. We see this today in our globalized world as we rely heavily on skills and goods from other parts of the world. Although both Weber and Durkheim wrote about the division of labor, Durkheim was more optimistic about it. He felt that the division of labor brings greater productivity and greater diversity, which could propel people toward exchange and perhaps greater unity. Unlike other scholars, he did not think that economics was entirely the key, but rather the social connectedness. He concluded that social order and individual autonomy were compatible.[8]

The major criticisms of this work, from today's perspective are many. First, when referring to individuals, Durkheim was referring to men, and did not include women in his conceptualization. Secondly, Durkheim differentiated industrialized from nonindustrialized without considering the possibility that societies may have characteristics of social solidarity.[6] Third, Durkheim overstated repressive law. He was basing his inferences on the Torah and early Christian Europe and appeared ignorant of the ethnographic literature.[22] Lastly, Durkheim's notion of a self-regulating division of labor exposed all the evils of unregulated capitalism but was remarkably uncritical of it.[24]

In *Elementary Forms of Religion,*[11] his most nuanced book, he examines the relationship of morality to religion. His theoretical lens is through the study of a "primitive" culture. In this study of an Australian clan, he articulates totemism as the most basic religion. The totem is the material representation of the conscious collective morality of the group. His premise was that in understanding the most basic or undifferentiated religious forms, the elements of social life gradually differentiated. In studying this single Australian clan, he made his most fundamental contributions concerning the symbolic nature of the sacred, theory of ritual, and role of religion in the internalization of values.[1] He posits that among all faiths (even the most secular), distinguish between divine and profane.[39] Ceremonies and rituals exemplify the divine; they are what morally binds people to their group or society. Morality is the glue that maintains a coherent and cohesive society, yet it is not inborn. From early in life, children learn about the sacred by observing and taking part in ceremonies and church. Moral practices, rites, and the church become the cognitive and affective frame through which individuals view the world and are bound together socially. He postulated how collective representations come about and then how they can also have a reciprocal influence on social structures.

Morality is inculcated and must be maintained by moral education in some form. In *Evolution of Pedagogy,*[14] he reviews his perspective on the history of French education as first appearing in the church during the middle ages. He suggests that the fundamentals of Christian world perspective view school as a place for education of the total personality, a conception which still survives.[1] Durkheim links Protestantism to science and the rise of realistic education. Collective representations emerge from and reflect social stratum. These influence social development. Once collective representations are institutionalized externally in social structures, these continue to influence people despite social and cultural changes. Provided that the social system is status quo, the putative system of collective representations will not be questioned.

Morality as articulated in *Professional Ethics and Civic Morals*[16] is composed of order (discipline to contain egoistic tendencies), attachment (desire to be committed to a group), and autonomy (individual responsibility). It also includes ideals of humanity. The role of collective representations in the social process together with his conception of structural differentiation outlines his theory of social change. During the first world war, Durkheim was active in attempting to counter the German propaganda. He held that what is sacred for us is the nation insofar as it embodies the ideal of humanity. The exception is, of course, the German policy of extermination, which Durkheim believed to be immoral. In this way, Durkheim placed morality as a higher standard than either the nation or the individual. Related to this, Durkheim admired some aspects of American Pragmatism but did not wholly believe in complete social construction of reality, as he saw this as a threat to rationalism. He believed that truth and reality had an objective moral character.

In his later writings, Durkheim emphasized the importance of history in understanding movements in social life. He emphasized the importance of studying more than simply the present perspective in order to understand the present as this may be influenced by existing urgencies and needs and passions of the present. As he stated in *Education and Sociology*, "...in order to know ourselves well, it is not enough to direct our attention to the superficial portion of our consciousness; for the sentiments, the ideas which come to the surface are not, by far, those which have the most influence on our conduct. What must be reached are the habits, the tendencies which have been established gradually in the course of our past life or which hereditary has bequeathed us; these are the real forces which govern us. Now, they are concealed in the unconscious. We can, the, success in discovering them only by reconstructing our personal history and the history of our family...(similarly) only history can penetrate under the surface of our present education system; only history can analyze it; only history...can bring us to the long chain of causes and effects of which it is the result".[1,14] This should be familiar to psychoanalysts of today as he was advocating a sociological analog to the psychoanalytic method to further understand a current social fact.[1]

CURRENT STATUS

Perhaps the prime legacy that Durkheim left is the importance that society has on individual mental health. While few can deny the recent neurobiological connections to individuals' various psychiatric symptoms, a person's cognitions, affects, and behaviors cannot be reduced to individual psychological factors. Society influences the individual in major ways by providing social purpose and ideals, rules and rituals for connection, and moral values to modify their desires. Within a society, or group, people are influenced by collective representations which are not reducible to individuals which dictate the ways in which individuals relate to one another.

Durkheim posited that, in his contemporary society, the personality had become sacred. "The modern system of collective consciousness" is the cult of the individual. Durkheim argued that "egoism, or the selfish pursuit of individual interests, is at odds with moral individualism, the ability to sacrifice self-interest for the rights of all other individuals".[39]

Our current world, advancing far beyond Durkheim's society, has continued to develop technological advances. These influence the impact that norms, laws, and culture have on the social integration of the community.

In contemporary empirical language we refer to these notions as social cohesion and social capital, which is the capacities of individuals to draw on collective resources of the group. There is a vast literature that supports that social capital and social cohesion is protective of mental health.[20] In a large study across four countries (Ethopia, India, Vietnam, and Peru), De Silva and colleagues (2007)[7] found that social capital reduces the risk of utilizing community mental health services.

Social fragmentation, which includes the erosion of a set of norms, and increased anonymity, is associated with urbanization and inner city life.[4] We see when there is erosion of common values over time, anomie increases. Durkheim's notions of the erosion of integration and regulation occur with the inevitable advancement of technology and urbanization. There are many studies that show that social fragmentation particularly in urban settings is associated with higher rates of schizophrenia, personality and impulse disorders, and depression.[4] The exception is that suicide is increased in rural areas, which may relate to lack of social networks and social isolation. While no doubt individual attention to those in the community who suffer with these conditions may require some individual intervention, the use of community resources to build greater neighborhood community may alleviate some of pressure on the mental health system.

Many of our urban areas have a multitude of ethnic communities. Migrant workers may experience more intensely. Language barriers and law of custom familiarity can lead to social isolation with increased mental health difficulties.[4] If, however, there is a larger community from the same ethnic background, these may protect minorities. An empirical study found that a higher ethnic density reduces mental health issues in African Americans and Hispanics.[38] This would suggest that communities that offer diverse support groups may alleviate the psychological distress and social isolation. The fostering of group identity has been noted as a protective factor in disorders such as post-traumatic stress disorder (PTSD).[25]

When there are sudden changes in the environment, our social structures and social order may be thrown into chaos. For instance, during the global pandemic of COVID, the requirement of lockdown created an environment where previous social structures and norms were unclear and unstable. Social isolation was inevitable. There was much conflict among groups who wanted to preserve the social order of social interaction and those who felt that fear of the illness and death dictated the isolation. The pandemic highlighted the visibility of anomie as there was a weakening of the previously established social bonds.[32] As predicted, there were increased suicides and death by overdose.[3] However, in the process, a new social order was created relying on technology. There was a springing up of virtual psychiatry visits, online classes, and webinars. Many who felt the use of technology in this were surprised at its effectiveness. Skill in technology and having online availability created the new order in the way that Durkheim has described.[32] We saw in psychiatry that those without those social resources were particularly disadvantaged and at risk for further separation from their peer groups. Children from poorer areas without computer availability remain still at risk in terms of cognitive and social development. We should expect to see in our offices for years to come the sequelae from this pandemic. The use of group could be particularly helpful in helping with relational development particularly in children and adolescents.

Sudden natural and manmade disasters can lead instability in the group. Immigrant communities are particularly vulnerable. Social support has been found to reduce PTSD symptoms. For example, in a longitudinal study with Vietnamese New Orleanians after Hurricane Katrina, social support provided soon after the event was positively associated with mental health even 4 years later.[23] One's perception of the social support is more relevant than the specific support given. Those people who perceive help with social supports are likely to suffer less. A study after Hurricane Sandy showed that those who have a positive regard for social support (e.g., hospitals and medical providers) prior to the disaster tend to have better mental health outcomes.[2] Perceiving social structures in a supportive light can serve as a buffer in times of disaster. Psychiatry would do well to augment their organizations and structures with the community so that if a disaster occurs supportive psychiatry is seen as a social fact.

Durkheim in his discussion of mechanical and organic societies provides an interesting perspective on understanding the upheaval apparent within societies and between them.[8] In a mechanical society, single conscious collective guides all. In a differentiated society where division of labor becomes important, the sphere of conscious collective has diminished. There is greater individual variation afforded by a diverse society. While technology and desire for individual thought allow for growth. Groups struggling to make the changes in demographics and diverse labor opportunities may long for the simpler life where all agree on the same. For example, far right conservative groups in the US long for a simpler, fundamental religious society where all would participate versus the more secular view of a freedom for the practice of all religions. In this later group, there is a breakdown of the integration of connections and a shared collective consciousness in the insistence of a moral set of values versus the freedom to pursue individual variations of human existence in terms of gender, sexuality, religious, cultural, and health practices.

Similarly, in our world, we have nations in various stages of the continuum between a mechanical solidarity and an organic solidarity. With different social structures, laws, norms, and culture, we see the tension between the characteristics of each society that clash between the countries—this is often along the demarcation of developed and developing countries. Here, both the restitutive and penal laws may clash and the efforts are made to collaborate by the use of treaties and coalitions of nations espousing to the same values.

CONCLUDING REMARKS

Émile Durkheim a well-known French Sociologist is considered one of the founding members of modern sociology. He is credited with making sociology a science through his application of scientific and empirical research. He proposed several notable sociological concepts: Mechanical and organic solidarity; collective conscious representation, "social facts" as a *sui generis*, and anomie and suicide. Most important legacy that Durkheim left psychiatry is the importance that society has on individual mental health and recognition that these connections are necessary for physical and emotional survival and health.

REFERENCES

1. Bellah R. Durkheim and history. Am Soc Rev. 1959;24(4):447-61.
2. Ben-Ezra M, Goodwin R, Palgi Y, Kaniasty K, Crawford MZ, Weinberger A, et al. Concomitants of perceived trust in hospital and medical services following Hurricane Sandy. Psychiatry Res. 2014;220(3):1160-2.
3. Bridge J, Ruch D, Sheftall A, Hahm C, O'Keefe V, Fontanella C, et al. Youth Suicide During the First Year of the COVID-19 Pandemic. Pediatrics. 2023;151(3):e2022058375.
4. Burns J. Psychosocial determinants of mental disorders. In: Burns J, Roos L (Eds). Textbook of Psychiatry for Southern Africa, 2nd Edition. Cape Town: Oxford University Press Southern Africa; 2016. pp. 72-90.
5. Crossman A. (2019). Understanding Durkheim's Division of Labor Views on Social Change and the Industrial Revolution. [online] Available from https://www.thoughtco.com/mechanical-solidarity-3026761. [Last accessed February, 2025]
6. De Silva M, Huttly S, Harpham T, Kenward M. Social capital and mental health: a comparative analysis of four low-income countries. Soc Sci Med. 2007;64(1): 5-20.
7. Durkheim, Émile. The Division of Labor in Society: A Study of the Organization of Higher Societies. Paris: Felix Alcan, 1893.
8. Durkheim, Émile. The Rules of Sociological Method. Paris: Felix Alcan, 1895.
9. Durkheim, Émile. Suicide: A Study in Sociology. Paris: Felix Alcan, 1897.
10. Durkheim, Émile. The Elementary Forms of the Religious Life: The Totemic System in Australia. Paris: Felix Alcan, 1915.
11. Durkheim, Émile. Education and Sociology. Paris: Felix Alcan, 1922.
12. Durkheim, Émile. Moral Education. Paris: Felix Alcan, 1925.
13. Durkheim, Émile. The Evolution of Educational Thought in France. 1938.
14. Durkheim, Émile. Sociology and Philosophy. Preface by Celestin Bouglé. Paris: Felix Alcan, 1924.
15. Durkheim É. (Lectures delivered 1890-1900). Professional Ethics and Civic Morals. Translated by Kennedy AG. Los Angeles: The Free Press; 1957.

16. Guyer JI. The true gift: Thoughts on L'Année sociologique of 1925. Journal of Classical Sociology. 2014;14(1):11-21. https://doi.org/10.1177/1468795X 13494714
17. Harpham T, Grant E, Thomas E. Measuring social capital within health surveys: Key issues. Health Policy Plan. 2002;17(1):106-11.
18. Haw C, Hawton K, Niedzwiedz C, Platt S. Suicide clusters: a review of risk factors and mechanisms. Suicide Life Threat Behav. 2013;43(1):97-108.
19. Jones R. Emile Durkheim: An Introduction to Four Major Works. London: Sage Publications; 1986.
20. Bui BKH, Anglewicz P, VanLandingham MJ. The impact of early social support on subsequent health recovery after a major disaster: a longitudinal analysis. SSM Popul Health. 2021;14:100779.
21. Lukes S. Emile Durkheim: His Life and Work. New York: Harper & Row Publishers; 1972.
22. Lyons M, Buhaol D, Fallon A. Trauma and Trauma Disorders. In: Gogineni R, Pumariega A, Kallivayalil R, Kastrup M, Rothe E (Eds). The WASP Textbook on Social Psychiatry: Historical, Developmental, Cultural and Clinical Perspectives. US: Oxford University Press; 2023.
23. Marson S. Elder Suicide: Durkheim's vision. North Carolina: NASW Press; 2019.
24. Mueller A, Abrutyn S, Pescosolido B, Diefendorf S. The social roots of suicide: Theorizing how the external social world matters to suicide and suicide prevention. Front Psychol. 2021;12:1-14.
25. Pattanaik N. (2021). Pandemic and Society: From the Durkheimian Lens. [online] Available from https://thesociologicalreview.org/magazine/june-2021/sociological-theories/pandemic-and-society/. [Last accessed February, 2025]
26. Peyre HM. (2024). Émile Durkheim. [online] Available from https://www.britannica.com/biography/Emile-Durkheim. [Last accessed February, 2025]
27. Ramp W. The Moral Discourse of Durkheim's Suicide. In: Pickering W, Walford G (Eds). Durkheim's Suicide: A Century of Research and Debate. Oxfordshire: Taylor and Francis Group; 2000. pp. 81-96.
28. Shaw R, Atkin K, Bécares L, Albor CB, Stafford M, Kiernan K, et al. Impact of ethnic density on adult mental disorders: a narrative review. Br J Psychiatry. 2012;201(1):11-9.
29. Smith T. (1984). Iran: Five Years of Fanaticism. [online] Available from https://www.nytimes.com/1984/02/12/magazine/iran-five-years-of-fanaticism.html. [Last accessed February, 2025]
30. Varty J. Suicide, Statistics and Sociology: Assessing Douglas' critique of Durkheim. In: Pickering W, Walford G (Eds). Durkheim's Suicide: A Century of Research and Debate. Oxfordshire: Taylor and Francis Group; 2000. pp. 53-65.
31. Peyre, H. (2025). Emile Durkheim: French Social Scientist. Britannica Retrieved Feb 25/25 https://www.britannica.com/biography/Emile-Durkheim
32. Hurst, A. (2023). Biography of Emile Durkheim. Retrieved 2/23/25 https://socialsci.libretexts.org/Bookshelves/Sociology/Introduction_to_Sociology/Classical_Sociological_Theory_and_Foundations_of_American_Sociology_(Hurst)/02%3A_Durkhcim/2.01%3A_Biography_of_Durkheim
33. Mestas, M. & Arendt, F. (2022). Suicide reporting in the nineteenth century: Large-Scale Descriptive Content Analysis of Austrian Newspapers. Media History, 29, 1-16.

34. Besnard, P. (2000). The Fortunes of Durkheim's Suicide: Reception and legacy. In In W. Pickering & G Walford (Eds.). Durkheim's Suicide: A Century of Research and Debate. Pp. 97-114, Taylor and Francis Group.
35. Besnard, P. (1983). The sociological domain: The durkheimians and the founding of French sociology. Cambridge, Cambridge University Press.
36. Joiner, T. (2005). Why People Die by Suicide: Massachusetts: Harvard University Press.
37. Lester, B. (2001). Learnings from Durkheim and Beyond: The Economy and Suicide Suicide and Life-Threatening Behavior 31(1) 15-31.
38. Lukes, S. (1972). Emile Durkheim: His Life and Work. Harper & Rox Publisher, New York.
39. Malik, H. & Malik, F. (2022). Emile Durkheim Contributions to Sociology. International Journal of Academic Multidisciplinary Research, 6, 7-10.

Theodor W Adorno

Jyoti M Rao

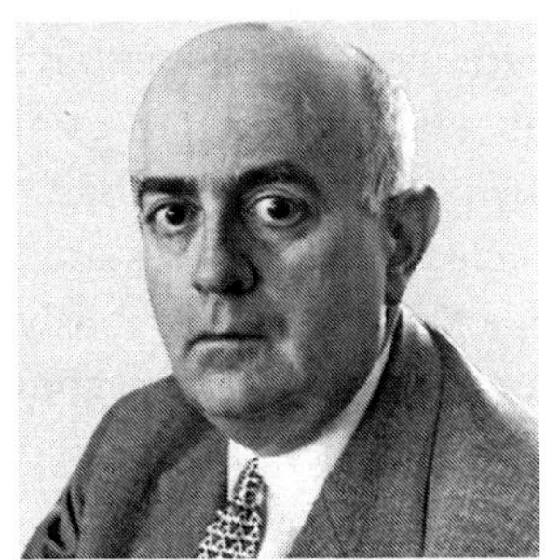

(1903–1969)

INTRODUCTION

Theodor Adorno was a profoundly interdisciplinary social theorist, whose work demonstrates the richness facilitated by refusing the intellectual balkanization that characterizes contemporary academic and clinical training. At the age of 21, Adorno completed doctoral research that mingled philosophy, musicology, psychology, and sociology.[1] He would synthesize these disciplines and more to creatively consider large-scale social questions, including authoritarianism, prejudice, emancipatory potentials, political ideology, and the nature of culture and cultural productions. A member of the Frankfurt School, he and his colleagues carefully theorized the most pressing and damaging societal dynamics of their time, many of which continue in our time, rooted as they are in persistent features of social and psychological life. The scholarly investigations of Adorno also demonstrate the wide-ranging nature of psychoanalytic inquiry that encompasses individuals as well as societal and cultural phenomena, recalling the primary, notably unrestricted, definition of psychoanalysis provided by Freud as a method of investigating mental processes that are made largely inaccessible because they are obscured from direct, conscious awareness.[2] Much as a psychoanalytic clinician attends to the invisible and unacknowledged undergirding of an analysand's psychic structure, e.g., in an individual who plainly undermines their own consciously desired contentment; Adorno labored at understanding the aspects of social experience that are hidden in plain sight, studying, among

TABLE 1: Notable publications.

- Dialectic of Enlightenment (1947)
- The Authoritarian Personality (1950)
- "Freudian Theory and the Pattern of Fascist Propaganda" (1951)
- Minima Moralia (1951)
- "On the Relationship between Sociology and Psychology" (1955)
- Negative Dialectics (1966)

other topics, the ways in which democratic societies hold self-destructive elements that periodically erupt in catastrophic ways. Adorno informs us that we are constantly acted upon and shaped by societal forces that are in dynamic and unconscious relationship with us as individuals and groups. In a structure that might be pictured as a mobile with interlinked parts, our individual, dyadic, and societal experiences are in constantly fluctuating, mutually influencing interaction both consciously and unconsciously, with important ramifications for the integrated psychoanalytic understanding of subjective life.[3] As we will see, Adorno posits specific ideas about the relative placement of the individual, psychological, and sociopolitical, especially as these relate to authoritarianism and fascism. This chapter will offer an overview of Adorno's life and extensive scholarship, including a discussion of the enduring importance of his ideas.

BRIEF BIOGRAPHY

Before embarking on this biographical sketch of Adorno's life, it must be noted that Adorno was highly critical of the social function of biographies, believing them to be largely fictional constructions trafficking in ideas of false coherence, linearity, the absence of ambivalence, and claims to truth that are vulnerable to being exploited as a tool of indoctrination.[4] In Adorno's words,[4] "At bottom, the concept of life as a meaningful unity unfolding from within itself has ceased to possess any reality, much like the individual himself, and the ideological function of biographies consists in demonstrating to people with reference to various models that something like life still exists, with all the emphatic qualities of life." A central preoccupation in Adorno's work is the numerous ways society encourages substituting 'something like life' for the insurgent vitality of life itself, a danger about which he demonstrates great vigilance. Adorno's stance of skepticism is an ethos congruent with the hermeneutics of suspicion attributed to Freud, Marx, and others whose ideas he engaged with. Composing a chapter on Adorno—or outlining his biographical details—without exhorting the reader to read critically toward the social function of such a text would be an omission that would be an injustice to Adorno's thinking.

Theodor Ludwig Wiesengrund, later to be known as Theodor W Adorno, was born on September 11, 1903. He was an only child in a wealthy family with a mixed cultural and religious background. His father was German of Jewish heritage, and had converted to Protestantism; his Corsican Catholic mother, from whose family name he would eventually take *Adorno,* was once a professional singer and introduced Adorno to music at a young age. Adorno's love of music performance and composition, as well as his study of musicology, would remain with him throughout his life. He began reading philosophy as a teenager and studied it with literary editor Siegfried Kracauer; the correspondence between the two men over the decades reveals an enduring intellectual and emotional intimacy with marked erotic elements.[5] As a young adult in the 1920s, Adorno would publish scholarly reviews of concerts in German language journals, and studied music intensively as he pursued his doctoral work in philosophy. Grounded in a critique of ideology that had already taken hold in his intellectual development, Adorno would use his specialized knowledge of music as a launching point for interdisciplinary insights into the wider social totality, combining "musicological analysis and sociological investigations of both the ways society shapes music and the public impacts of its production, reception, and distribution".[1]

Adorno met many of his future collaborators, including Max Horkheimer and Walter Benjamin, in the 1920s; their generation would see the ravages of both World Wars and the societal disarray that preceded and followed those tragedies. In the summer of 1924, Adorno completed his doctorate in philosophy, and moved to Vienna the following year. There, he studied composition, piano, violin, and attended public lectures; his musical works would be performed in Vienna as his work in philosophy began in earnest. One of his first works, entitled "The Concept of the Unconscious in the Transcendental Theory of the Psyche," explored Freud's emerging theories of the unconscious. By the end of the 1920s and in the beginning of the 1930s, Adorno worked toward an academic post in philosophy, which he acquired in 1931. Around this time, he delivered his first talk at the Institute for Social Research, launching his lifelong involvement with what would be known as the Frankfurt School. Within a few years, his academic position, and indeed, his entire life in Europe, would be upended by Nazi power. Adorno began a life of exile, first in the UK, where he moved in 1934 to study at Oxford; then to the United States in 1938. He would marry his wife, Margarete "Gretel" Karplus, with whom he had been in an often long-distance relationship for over a decade, in 1937. Gretel Karplus Adorno, who held a doctorate degree in chemistry and was a manager of a factory, had an unsung role in Adorno's life work, working at the Institute for Social Research, and serving as "Adorno's confidant, companion, secretary, manager, editor, and buffer to the outside world".[6] Horkheimer and Adorno acknowledge her "valuable assistance" in "continuing to develop their theory" in their prefaces to *Dialectic of Enlightenment.*[7]

The linguistic and cultural displacement experienced by Adorno upon his exile to the US, the alienating sequelae of which are reported by him in his highly personal work *Minima Moralia,* is congruent with contemporary psychoanalytic literature on the trauma of immigration and displacement. Much of his scholarly work may be considered through the lens of his perpetual status as an outsider, which provided him a lens from which the workings of culture became visible. While McLaughlin[8] coined the phrase "optimal marginality" to consider the role of marginality in Erik Fromm's innovative thinking, one might equally contemplate experiences of social marginality in formatively shaping Adorno's subjectivity and the novel insights it yielded. Adorno lived and worked in the United States from the late 1930s until 1949, when Adorno returned to Frankfurt and began with others to rebuild the school of critical theory they had been a part of when Hitler came to power. Between 1941 and 1948, he codirected the Research Project on Social Discrimination at the University of California at Berkeley; this work would be compiled in *The Authoritarian Personality*, published in 1950. After his return to Germany, he would continue the work of analyzing the rise and fall of the Nazi regime, which he felt was not an isolated event but rather a tendency within societies that could repeat. He published *Freudian Theory and the Pattern of Fascist Propaganda* in 1951. After being appointed as full professor of sociology and philosophy at the University of Frankfurt in 1956, he was co-appointed as director of the revived Institute for Social Research in Frankfurt in 1958.

During the two decades following his return to Germany in the early 1950s, Adorno would establish himself as an influential public intellectual and academic, writing and speaking prolifically in the areas of social psychology, political theory, philosophy, music, and cultural criticism. His lectures were influential and well-attended until the end of his life. Among Adorno's most well-known students are the German social philosopher Jürgen Habermas and American political activist, philosopher, and academic Angela Davis, who studied first with Herbert Marcuse in the United States, then with Adorno in Germany in the 1960s. During the height of the student protest movement, Marcuse and Adorno would exchange letters debating the role of student protest and the use of police force against students.[9] Adorno died in 1969 of a heart attack in Switzerland. In part because his works in German were largely untranslated at the time of his death, the New York Times ran an obituary that was remarkable in its inadequate representation of the significance of Adorno's life work.[10] In 1997, a 20-volume edition of collected works by Adorno was released in German.

MAJOR CONTRIBUTIONS

A succinct summary of Adorno's theoretical contributions is a formidable, and indeed, impossible task for numerous reasons. First, his enormous body of work is embedded in a sophisticated intellectual history, including longstanding debates within continental philosophy which are outside of the scope of this chapter. *Dialectic of Enlightenment* and *Negative Dialectics* are major philosophical works by Adorno within this tradition, among others. In addition, Adorno addressed an impressive range of subject matter with depth across diverse disciplines, including musicology and cultural studies, that cannot be discussed here even briefly. His critique of the culture industry, e.g. in which he considered the role of television, film, and other media, comprises an essential element of his thinking, and should be investigated by anyone interested in learning more about Adorno's work. This section will touch on only two key aspects of Adorno's work: the concept of critical theory and Adorno's work on authoritarianism and fascism. What appears below is not intended as a comprehensive overview of Adorno's weighty offerings on these two topics, much less the remainder of his voluminous theoretical corpus; it stands only as a springboard for the further study of the interested reader. Adorno and his Frankfurt School colleagues were committed to using psychoanalytic insights together with philosophy and social science in the service of emancipatory potentials;[10] this thread, woven throughout Adorno's work, will be highlighted below.

Critical Theory

The work of the Frankfurt School theorists, including Adorno, worked toward theorizations of society and culture that built on the thinking of Freud, Marx, philosophers such as Hegel, sociologists, and scholars in other allied disciplines; it is explicitly anticapitalist and has a social reform agenda aimed at the common good. The theory of Adorno and the Frankfurt School is termed *critical theory*. *Critical* here is in contrast to *traditional* theory, which are differentiated in a seminal essay by Adorno's long-term collaborator Max Horkheimer.[11] Horkheimer delineates that the aim of critical theory is to critique and change the very foundations of social reality to undertake "the abolition of social injustice." The inquiry undertaken within traditional theory operates within the existing social order, furthering dominant narratives and power structures in ways that are inherently conserving of the status quo, but mostly invisible to the traditional researcher. Crucially, critical theory holds within it a reflexive, self-analyzing function, perpetually interrogating the hidden forms of ideology and power it might be unintentionally propagating, reifying, and inhabiting.

For example, a psychiatric approach that focuses on the neurochemical aspects of depression embodies what Horkheimer might term *traditional* theory. As such, the medical perspective holds many unarticulated assumptions: that depression may be objectively perceived, quantified, and biomedically assessed on the individual level (likely excluding or minimizing the subjective, social, economic, and cultural dimensions of depression);

that the person or system conducting such an assessment may be neutral (overlooking the biases and social influences within which each person and system are necessarily embedded); and that the symptom of depression can and should be alleviated (potentially removing the depressed mood before its communicative significances and meanings may be comprehended). The medical position leaves unquestioned the terms and structures within which such a conceptualization of depression exists, and leaves unexamined the sociopolitical agendas such a framing might serve. Placed within traditional theory, the medical ecosystem largely exempts itself from these inquiries, and its practitioners are not trained to subject their actions and institutions to this form of scrutiny.

From a critical theory perspective, the very attempt to study the neurochemical aspects of depression would be problematized and critically examined: How does such a theorization of depressed mood serve existing conceptualizations of the self, society, government, and culture? If depressed mood exists as a form of resistance against capitalist (or patriarchal or racial or imperialist or other forms of) domination—e.g., by rendering one unable to go to one's exploitative workplace—does an emphasis on brain chemistry attempt to erase such resistance, reinscribing its sole meaning as chemical aberration within the individual's medicalized physical body? How does the biomedical conceptualization of depression act to render invisible central social factors that might generate dysphoria, such as poverty, prejudice, labor conditions, the alienation generated by commercialism, political persecution, and other forms of injustice? How might focusing on an individual's mood in medical terms prevent the formation of political groups that might discover newfound power through solidarity? How does psychiatry, and the medical institutions within which it is practiced and taught, promote a view of depression that reifies existing social arrangements, undermines critical analysis, and opposes change? Critical theory places these queries at its center, theorizing itself and its social placements even as it theorizes human experience in terms of social justice and injustice.

In accordance with this perspective, Adorno was critical of those who espoused a clinical psychoanalysis aimed at creating a "well-adjusted" person; he was especially troubled by this thread he perceived in Karen Horney's work, which he saw as inescapably allied with social conformity and pathogenic accommodation.[12] In his critique of Horney, Erik Erikson, and others who were working toward a more socially informed psychoanalysis in the United States, Adorno strongly opposed the move away from libido theory and the tendency to see alignment with the reality principle as potentially beneficial to the subject, rather than as an inherently violent capitulation to unjust and oppressive social norms. Adorno[13] writes that "on theoretical grounds," he disagrees with "attempts to 'sociologize' psychoanalysis through softening of basic concepts—e.g., the unconscious, infantile sexuality, the psychological dynamism of the monad—by looking for environmental influences which would have to be registered in terms of the ego rather than the unconscious." Such a psychoanalysis, in Adorno's view, promotes a clinical practice that unthinkingly herds the patient toward alliance with the interests of industrialized mass culture. The assumption of an autonomous subject separable from its social milieu, integral to many conceptions of psychoanalysis, was deeply suspect to Adorno, who felt that contemporary conditions created a fusion between the psyche and "social standardization" that rendered individual resistance elusive.[14] As Nilsson[12] summarizes Adorno's position:

> *If one is to adhere to the notion of the unconscious present in Freud's work—as Adorno and Horkheimer do—the belief in the unity of an individual's psychic life—and of a psychic unity of the human—whether conditioned by society or not, is undermined as the unconscious continually surfaces in opposition to the subject's conscious desire and the reality principle.*
>
> *Even though the Freudian unconscious is key for Adorno and Horkheimer as is highlights the possibility for the psychic to undermine social relations, it is not an object which is cordoned off from influence and change. [...] In this sense, Adorno and Horkheimer cannot be understood as just adherents of the Freudian libido theory, but rather produce a corrective to the theory through introducing Historicization into psychoanalysis (p. 8).*

In other words, by emphasizing the role of the unconscious as an ungovernable force in dialectic with societal forces (the reality principle), the critical theory of Adorno and his colleagues views the unconscious as a vital current on the side of socially emancipatory potentials in its intrinsic disruptiveness. Contemporary psychoanalyst Barnaby B Barratt,[15] working in this tradition and formulating a *radical psychoanalysis*, has taken a similar position in advocating for a subversion of the "ideological commitments" of psychotherapeutic practice to promote the emergence of a liberatory psychoanalysis.

Authoritarianism and Fascism

At the time of his death, Adorno was best known in the United States for his work as a principal author of *The Authoritarian Personality*, despite it being somewhat of a departure from his work as a whole, especially in its "uneasy" attempt to pair critical theory with the empirical methods and survey techniques in vogue in the United States at the time.[10] In his introductory remarks to the final study report, which bear careful examination, Adorno[13] positions the study in the context of studies on prejudice, and underscores his view that "the ultimate source of prejudice has to be sought in social factors which are incomparably stronger than the 'psyche' of any one individual involved." In addition, he writes that although the study is in the subject of "social psychology," it is "in full harmony with psychoanalysis in its more orthodox, Freudian version," elaborating that the psychological conceptualizations informing the study "definitely belong to psychoanalysis."

This powerful endorsement of psychoanalysis and the study as being built on "orthodox, Freudian" bedrock, may be read as a reminder by Adorno to recall unconscious process while considering what may otherwise appear to be a more psychosociological study about manifest character. Indeed, he takes some pains to distinguish the study's theoretical grounding from "the sociological approach," which Adorno says, "makes prejudice seem harmless—a necessary evil of organized society—and perennial... interpreted as invariants of social organization rather than the consequence of exploitation and repression".[13] As in the example given above of the medical conceptualization of depression as primarily a biological event, Adorno is concerned here about the naturalization of prejudice as an endemic, passively generated feature of taken-for-granted social dynamics, which may cause an investigator to fail in critically examining its active generation through oppressive structural underpinnings, and the identificatory processes that shape human behavior. Adorno clearly wishes the reader of *The Authoritarian Personality* to understand it through the lens of critical theory, contextualizing it with a vigilant stance and keeping psychoanalytic principles in mind.

The study itself was a joint project between the Institute for Social Research, led by Adorno, and the Berkeley Public Opinion Study, led by R Nevitt Sanford; it was supported by grants from the American Jewish Committee.[13] The other two principal researchers were the Polish refugee psychoanalyst Else Frenkel-Brunswik who was a research associate; and Daniel Levinson, who was then a graduate student at UC Berkeley and would later be a professor of psychology.[14] Sanford would be among those who were fired for refusing to sign McCarthy era anticommunist loyalty oaths; he and a number of his colleagues would be reinstated after winning a legal case in 1952 (Adorno had returned to Germany by this time).[16] The researchers emphasized the "thoroughly collective" nature of their work, perhaps in an attempt to model a collaborative sensibility. Their work was centered not on those who espoused fascistic ideas or belonged to fascist organizations, but rather on "the *potentially fascistic* individual, one whose structure is such as to render him particularly susceptible to antidemocratic propaganda".[13] Based on questions that arose in Nazi Germany about the ways in which the public was readily recruited toward fascism, this research was seeking answers about the patterns, shaped by political, economic, and social convictions, that might express "deep-lying trends" toward fascism in the personality.

The study entailed the development of a survey instrument administered to over 2,000 study participants. The design originally measured four scales, intended to capture antisemitism, ethnocentrism, politico-economic conservative ideological commitment, and the so-called "F scale," designed to assess potential for fascism (the conservative ideological commitment measure would be put aside for reasons of poor correlation).[14] The F scale was designed around Adorno's conceptualization of the features of authoritarianism, which included nine characteristics: conventionalism, authoritarian submission, authoritarian aggression, anti-intraception (a hostility to the imaginative, subjective, and "tender-minded"), superstition/stereotypic thinking, power and "toughness," destructiveness/ cynicism, projectivity, and an "exaggerated concern" with matters pertaining to sex.[13,14] The aim was to generate a profile of dormant features within the personality that, once exposed to a certain set of social conditions, was likely to veer into fascism. The researchers concluded that those in the small percentage who scored high on all scales were likely to be prejudiced against religious and cultural minorities including immigrants, Black Americans, and Jewish Americans, and hold conservative positions on issues pertaining to labor and welfare; this personality type, the authoritarian personality, was seen to hold the ready potential to express fascism.[13,15]

Some[14] have surmised that Adorno tempered his more radical perspectives in order to collaborate with his American colleagues—Adorno and his fellow Frankfurt School thinkers had categorical critiques of contemporary society itself, believing late capitalist society to have the seeds of authoritarianism deeply embedded within it. These views were somewhat subordinated to the conclusions of the study as outlined in *The Authoritarian Personality*, which undertook a psychological study of politics that focused on individual personality traits, and posited fascism as a political manifestation of dormant authoritarian features in the personality.[13]

Only a year after publishing *The Authoritarian Personality,* Adorno published the essay "Freudian Theory and the Pattern of Fascist Propaganda," in which he seems to correct the position taken in *The Authoritarian Personality.*[14] Historian Peter Gordon's[14] analysis of Adorno's positions in these two contrasting works quotes Adorno in "Freudian Theory and the Pattern of Fascist Propaganda":

> *For Adorno the AP-Study [Authoritarian Personality Study] had mistakenly reversed the directionality of causation in its theory of fascism. Rather than affirming the authoritarian personality as the actual* source *of its appeal, Adorno insisted that an authoritarian "character" be seen as the* introjection *of an irrational society. "Psychological dispositions do not actually cause fascism," Adorno*

> *explained. "Rather, fascism defines a psychological area which can be successfully exploited by the forces which promote it for entirely nonpsychological reasons of self-interest." (p. 64)*

In the essay on fascist propaganda, Adorno uses Freud's *Group Psychology* to consider the fascist crowd and its narcissistic identification with the leader, while simultaneously contending that fascism is not a phenomenon of the individual psyche and its psychology.[17] Adorno further outlines the "artificial regression" characteristic of rallies and other forms of fascistic group experiences that allow participants to feel a sense of full participation even as their material conditions are entirely unchanged. Gordon[14] summarizes Adorno as follows:

> *In this analysis fascism becomes simultaneously truth* and *untruth: On the one hand, it holds out to the masses the promise of a collective release from the constraints of bourgeois civilization with its demand that all instinct (and perhaps especially violence) submit to a pathological repression. Condemning this repression as pathological, it presents itself as the "honest" or "forthright" acknowledgement of everything one is not supposed to say or do. On the other hand, it offers merely the* performance *of this release through the fantasy of an identification with a leader who offers* both *the experience of masochistic submission* and *the illusion that he is just like his followers. This is fascism's "social miracle," which, like all miracles, serves as a dream of redemption without providing any actual transformation from the social conditions of unhappiness. (pp. 66-67)*

CURRENT STATUS

Adorno's work was remarkably prescient, and continues to have great relevance to current questions of interest. The topic of authoritarianism and antidemocratic processes are, of course, of central importance in contemplating the rise of present-day authoritarian global political figures; the fascistic workings that accompany their uses of power; and the public support for such figures, many of whom, like Adolf Hitler, are democratically elected. A roundtable held in 2017 at the New School of Social Research invited scholars to discuss Adorno's analysis of WWII era fascism in relationship to the politics of the present, especially in relationship to Donald Trump. In this series of presentations, Bernstein[18] states that Adorno's "Freudian Theory and the Pattern of Fascist Propaganda" reads "as if it was written precisely in order to address the Trump phenomenon," addressing as it does the narcissism of the leader who exploits the psychosocial function of social hatred of fabricated out-groups as a negative source of self-affirmation for the in-group. Bottici[17] applies the same text to the dynamics of group and leader in relationship to Trump, adding an important critique of the danger of naturalizing Eurocentric values when applying both Freud and Adorno to global societies, including in the multicultural US context. Examples of robust applications of Adorno in non-Euro-American contexts are found in Nandy's[19] study of fascism in India; Guohua and Xiangchun's study[20] of mass culture theory to the world of contemporary Chinese cultural criticism; and de Souza's[21] examination of present-day political radicalization in Brazil.

Gordon,[14] whose work was cited earlier in this chapter, takes an Adorno-centered analysis of the ascendency of Trump, suggesting it is best understood not merely as a function of an authoritarian personality or a regressive society, but rather as a function of the culture industry, which propagates the status quo even as it creates the pretense of undoing repression with high-stimulus public spectacles and vulgarity. Other recent works[22] have revisited psychological and societal aspects of authoritarianism in relationship to ideology and prejudice. While these scholars are continuing the political philosophy thread of Adorno's work, others are pursuing the social research Adorno began with *The Authoritarian Personality*, aimed at identifying fundamental, cross-culturally validated personality characteristics tied to authoritarianism. Research undertaken in 1974 replicated Adorno's model of studying of authoritarianism with subjects at the University of Punjab in India.[23] Using the scales formulated in the original study, but modifying the anti-Semitism measure to capture anti-Muslim sentiment, researchers translated the survey instrument into Hindi and Punjabi. The results of this study were almost identical to those of the Berkeley study, indicating cross-cultural consistency in authoritarian tendencies. More recently, Nai and Toros[24] studied global national leaders with autocratic tendencies, including Bolsonaro, Duterte, Erdoğan, Modi, Orbán, Netanyahu, Strache, and Trump among others; their findings showed that autocrats scored significantly higher on traits of narcissism, psychopathy, and Machiavellianism, and lower on traits of emotional stability and agreeableness.

Outside of the realm of politicians, many have sought out Adorno's understandings of historical transgressions to comprehend and ameliorate contemporary injustices. Some examples include formulating educational responses to the abuses of prisoners at Abu Ghraib,[25] noncompliance with public health recommendations in response to COVID-19,[26] anticapitalist political activism,[27] and social justice more broadly.[28,29] In the years following Adorno's death, his work has been extended and reexamined by multiple scholars. Many over the last few decades have sought to link Adorno's work with feminist theory and practice[30,31] as well as gender and queer theory,[32,33] including critiques of Adorno's thoughts on sexuality.[34] Peter Gordon's[35] current reading of Adorno emphasizes the sense of unfulfilled possibility embedded in Adorno's sometimes searing critique of social conditions; while it is important to comprehend what is damaged in society, its importance lies in the hope of realizing better potentials, which Gordon asserts is central to Adorno's theory. Nilsson's[12] reading of Adorno similarly highlights the desire for a society free of domination of self and other, a "real humanism."

Adorno's theorization about culture has spawned prolific academic work studying a range of cultural productions. Villarejo[36] considers Adorno's work on television in the contemporary context, addressing questions of psychosocial response, ideology, and capitalist inculcation, as well as representations of queer life.[37] Others[38-40] have considered Adorno's work in relationship to film studies; and music.[41,42] Adorno's comments on the popular appeal of astrology, including an analysis he conducted on the astrology column of the Los Angeles Times and the ideology of dependence he felt it generated, have gained new relevance in the contemporary moment, promoting scholars to revisit Adorno's theorization on the topic.[43]

CONCLUDING REMARKS

This chapter addresses the life and work of Theodor Adorno, a major theorist of the Frankfurt School. His prolific work was motivated by a desire to comprehensively theorize social conditions in the interest of promoting of social justice and more widespread social welfare. Adorno's scholarship is a model of interdisciplinarity, bringing together diverse approaches including philosophy, psychoanalysis, sociology, political theory, culture studies, and musicology to understand the nature of the world around us. The critical theory of Adorno and his collaborators encourages us to question everything, including the theory we study, the practices we undertake, and all of our suppositions about ourselves and the world we inhabit. For Adorno, this unceasing critical inquiry is required to comprehend and counter the determinants of authoritarianism and fascism, so that we may reclaim our capacities for resistance and not repeat the worst chapters of human history.

REFERENCES

1. Schweppenhäuser G. Theodor W. Adorno: An Introduction. Durham: Duke University Press; 2009.
2. Freud S. Two Encyclopaedia Articles. Standard Edition of the Complete Psychological Works of Sigmund Freud. London: Hogarth Press; Volume 18. 1923. pp. 235-59.
3. Rao JM. Social Justice Activism as Interpretation in a Loewaldian World. J Am Psychoanal Assoc. 2023;71:1149-73.
4. Claussen D. Theodor W. Adorno: One Last Genius. Cambridge: Harvard University Press; 2008.
5. von Moltke J. (2009). Teddie and Friedel: Theodor W. Adorno, Siegfried Kracauer, and the Erotics of Friendship. [online] Available from https://digitalcommons.wayne.edu/cgi/viewcontent.cgi?referer=&httpsredir=1&article=1579&context=criticism#:~:text=The%20two%20men's%20relation%2D%20ships,close%20of%20the%20letters%20have. [Last accessed February, 2025]

6. von Boekmann SL. (2004). The Life and Work of Gretel Karplus/Adorno: Her Contributions to Frankfurt School Theory. [online] Available from https://shareok.org/server/api/core/bitstreams/4f989737-955c-42fc-9f04-93528b2d929f/content. [Last accessed February, 2025]
7. Horkheimer M, Adorno TW, Noerr GS. Dialectic of Enlightenment: Philosophical Fragments. Stanford: Stanford University Press; 1987.
8. McLaughlin N. Optimal Marginality: Innovation and Orthodoxy in Fromm's Revision of Psychoanalysis. Sociol Quart. 2001;42:271-88.
9. Adorno TW, Marcuse H, Leslie E. (Trans.) Correspondence on the German Student Movement. N Left Rev. 1999;233:123-36.
10. Jay M. (1984). Adorno in America. [online] Available from https://www.jstor.org/stable/487894. [Last accessed February, 2025]
11. Horkheimer M, O'Connell MJ. (Trans.) Traditional and Critical Theory. In Critical Theory: Selected Essays. New York: Continuum; 1972.
12. Nilsson A. (2023). The humanism of critical theory: The Frankfurt School's 'realer humanismus'. [online] Available from https://journals.sagepub.com/doi/10.1177/01914537231170904?icid=int.sj-abstract.citing-articles.1#:~:text=Rather%2C%20the%20'Real%20Humanism',essence%20which%20must%20be%20freed. [Last accessed February, 2025]
13. Adorno TW, Frenkel-Brunswik E, Levinson DJ, Sanford RN. The Authoritarian Personality. London: Verso; 2019/1950.
14. Gordon P. The Authoritarian Personality Revisited. In Authoritarianism: Three Inquiries in Critical Studies. Chicago: University of Chicago Press; 2018.
15. Barratt BB. On Difference and the "Beyond Psychotherapy" of Psychoanalytic Method: The Pivotal Issue of Free-Associative Discourse as De-Repressive Praxis. Am J Psychoanal. 2021;81:27-50.
16. Roiser M, Willig C. The strange death of the authoritarian personality: 50 years of psychological and political debate. Hist Human Sci. 2002;15:71-96.
17. Bottici C. (2017). Adorno with Freud, Adorno Beyond Freud. [Roundtable Presentation] New School of Social Research (2017, October 5). [online] Available from https://publicseminar.org/2017/10/adorno-with-freud-adorno-beyond-freud/. [Last accessed February, 2025]
18. Bernstein J. (2017). Adorno's Uncanny Analysis of Trump's Authoritarian Personality. [Roundtable Presentation] New School of Social Research (2017, October 5). [online] Available from https://publicseminar.org/2017/10/adornos-uncanny-analysis-of-trumps-authoritarian-personality/. [Last accessed February, 2025]
19. Nandy A. Adorno in India: Revisiting the psychology of Fascism. Indian J Psychol. 1976;51:168-78.
20. Guohua Z, Xiangchun M. Chinese practice and T. W. Adorno's theory of mass culture. Neohelicon. 2014;41:489-502.
21. de Souza MR. Fascism in nowadays Brazil: On the topicality of Adorno's Education after Auschwitz. J Theor Philos Psychol. 2022;42:189-201.
22. Osborne D, Costello TH, Duckitt J, Sibley CG. The psychological causes and societal consequences of authoritarianism. Nat Rev Psychol. 2023;2:220-32.
23. Varma VK, Akhtar S, Kulhara PN, Kaushal P. Measurement of Authoritarian Traits in India. Indian J Psy. 1973;15:156-75.

24. Nai A, Toros E. The peculiar personality of strongmen: comparing the Big Five and Dark Triad traits of autocrats and non-autocrats. Polit Res Exchange. 2020;2:1-24.
25. Giroux HA. Education after Abu Ghraib: Revisiting Adorno's Politics of Education. Cult Studies. 2006;18:779-815.
26. Salone A, Ciavoni L, Di Muzio I, Santovito MC. Denial as a psychological process underlying non-compliance with public health recommendations for the prevention of COVID-19. J Ital Soc Psychiatry. 2021;7:134-40.
27. Holloway J, Matamoros F, Tischler S. Negativity and Revolution: Adorno and Political Activism. London: Pluto; 2009.
28. Kuebler F. 'Suffering ought not to be': Adorno on the dialectics of memory. Envir Plan F. 2023;2:421-37.
29. McArthur J. Rethinking knowledge within higher education: Adorno and social justice. London: Bloomsbury Academic; 2013.
30. Heberle RJ. Feminist Interpretations of Theodor Adorno. University Park: Penn State Press; 2006.
31. O'Neill M. Adorno, Culture, and Feminism. London: Sage Publications; 1999.
32. Duford R. Daughters of the Enlightenment: Reconstructing Adorno on Gender and Feminist Praxis. Hypatia. 2017;32:784-800.
33. Halle R. Queer Social Philosophy: Critical Readings from Kant to Adorno. Chicago: University of Illinois; 2004.
34. Halle R. Between Marxism and psychoanalysis: antifascism and anti-homosexuality in the Frankfurt School. J Homosex. 1995;29:295-317.
35. Gordon PE. A precarious happiness: Adorno and the sources of normativity. Chicago: University of Chicago Press; 2024.
36. Villarejo A. Adorno by the Pool; Or, Television Then and Now. Social Text. 2016;34:71-87.
37. Villarejo A. Ethereal Queer: Television, Historicity, Desire. Durham: Duke University Press; 2014.
38. D'Olimpio L. (2014). Thoughts on film: Critically engaging with both Adorno and Benjamin. [online] Available from https://www.tandfonline.com/doi/full/10.1080/00131857.2014.964161. [Last accessed February, 2025]
39. Hansen MB, Dimendberg E. Cinema and Experience: Siegfried Kracauer, Walter Benjamin, and Theodor W. Adorno. Berkeley: University of California Press; 2011.
40. Wall B. Theodor Adorno and Film Theory: The Fingerprint of Spirit. New York: MacMillan; 2013.
41. Engh B. Of Music and Mimesis. In: O'Neill M (Ed). Adorno, Culture, and Feminism. London: Sage Publications; 1999.
42. Steinberg MP. The Musical Absolute. N German Crit. 1992;56:17-42.
43. Nederman CJ, James WG. "Popular Occultism and Critical Social Theory: Exploring Some Themes in Adorno's Critique of Astrology and the Occult." Sociol Analys. 1981;42:325-32.

Social and Community Psychiatrists

8. **Joshua Bierer**
   Vincenzo Di Nicola, Rama Rao Gogineni
9. **George Morrison Carstairs**
   Mohan Isaac
10. **Norman Sartorius**
    Debasish Basu
11. **Ravi L Kapur**
    Roy A Kallivayalil, Rakesh K Chadda
12. **Julian Leff**
    Tom KJ Craig

CHAPTER 8

Joshua Bierer

Vincenzo Di Nicola, Rama Rao Gogineni

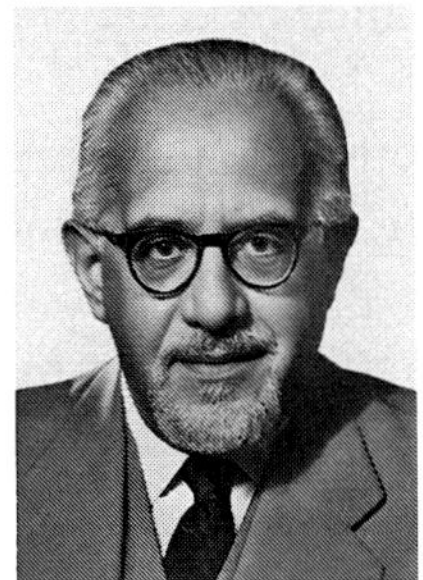

(1901–1984)

INTRODUCTION

Joshua Bierer, founder of Institute of Social Psychiatry in London, UK and the *International Journal of Social Psychiatry* 70 years ago, was a creative trailblazer who should be remembered as a dedicated clinician, organizer, philosopher of psychiatry, and above all, as a social psychiatrist for his contributions to understanding and promoting the *social* in psychiatry and mental health.[1] Trained in Austria with Alfred Adler, he practiced in Berlin, Germany, and Vienna, Austria before going to Britain to become the first consultant psychotherapist in a public mental hospital. Bierer was at the center of the key developments of his day in psychotherapy and social psychiatry which were central to his thinking as well as during his career in Europe and America.[1-6]

The World Association of Social Psychiatry (WASP) was founded in 1964 by Joshua Bierer of the UK and other like-minded people committed to the cause of social psychiatry. Initially, it was named as the *International Congress of Social Psychiatry* and at the 6th Congress (1974), it was renamed as the *World Association of Social Psychiatry*. Bierer was the organizer of the first three world congresses of Social Psychiatry. He was also the founding editor of the *International Journal of Social Psychiatry*, Founder and Chairman of the Institute of Social Psychiatry in London, and Founder and Chairman of the British Association of Social Psychiatry.[5] Bierer published extensively, in community care and rehabilitation of patients with chronic disabilities.

He was an enthusiastic lecturer, much in demand in the UK and abroad. He was one of the Jewish exiles from Austria and Nazi Germany who have enriched British psychiatry and contribute widely to its present status.[1]

BRIEF BIOGRAPHY

Joshua Bierer was born in Radautz, then part of Austria, now known as Rădăuţi in Romania, into a distinguished Jewish family in which all male members for three generations were medical doctors, his great grandfather was court physician to the King of Serbia and a great friend of Theodor Herzl, founder of the Zionist movement. He died in Tenerife on November 22, 1984, at the age of 83.[1]

After receiving his early education in Austria, Bierer trained in individual psychology with Alfred Adler, a student of Sigmund Freud who broke off from the main psychoanalytic movement to found his own school of individual psychology. This is an intriguing beginning since Bierer distinguished himself by situating psychiatry in a broader social context rather than Adler's individual approach. When he completed his training analysis, he was appointed to the Teaching Institute in Individual Psychology in Berlin in 1928.[1]

He began his career in psychotherapy working at various Austrian mental hospitals. At this time, he carried out pioneering work in psychotherapy at mental hospitals in Vienna and in 1938, he was awarded his MD. However, he was prompted by rising anti-Semitism to emigrate in the 1930s, first to what was then the British Mandate for Palestine and then to the UK, where he was appointed as the first psychotherapist at the recently opened Runwell Mental Hospital in 1938. He founded the first therapeutic community there. After a brief period as a clinical assistant at Guy's Hospital, he joined the Royal Army Medical Corps (RAMC) in which he served for most of the war. As a member of the RAMC, Bierer was, for a while, associated with the experiments taking place at the Northfield Military Neurosis Centre where he had established group psychotherapy in his own ward and in his own style.[1]

In 1946, Bierer founded a social psychotherapy center, named the Marlborough Day Hospital, which was the first hospital of this kind in the world[7] at the same time as Ewen Cameron at McGill University in Montreal, Canada.[8] He had many firsts to his credit: Founder and Editor of the International Journal of Social Psychiatry, Founder and Chairman of the Institute of Social Psychiatry, and Founder and Chairman of the British Association of Social Psychiatry. He published extensively, mainly in community care and rehabilitation of mental patients with chronic disabilities. Key papers included "Treatment of Psychotic Patients in Mental Hospitals," "Out-patient Psychotherapy," and with Professor RI Evans, "Innovations in Social Psychiatry".[1,2]

Bierer was working in the National Health Service of postwar Britain at a time of innovative developments in social psychiatry and social services in London itself and Britain overall[9] that were auspicious for a broader, more social view of psychiatry and mental health[10] with greater sensitivity to and recognition of social class,[11,12] anticipating the pioneering social epidemiology of the WHO Social Determinants of Health[13] and the US Adverse Childhood Experiences Study.[14] It was a time of moving out of institutions and into the community with bridging concepts and interventions like milieu therapy[15] and the therapeutic community.[16] Social stress was beginning to be defined and documented as a factor in mental illness.[17] Furthermore, society itself was seen as a patient[18] and mental hospitals were critiqued as "total institutions" using coercive measures.[19] All of this contributed to Bierer's impact and was part of the nascent community psychiatry and community mental health movement.[20]

Bierer was the founder and organizer of the first three world congresses of social psychiatry. He was also the founder editor of the *International Journal of Social Psychiatry*, Founder and Chairman of the Institute of Social Psychiatry, and Founder and Chairman of the British Association of Social Psychiatry.[21] He published extensively, in community mental health care and rehabilitation of patients with chronic disabilities. He was an enthusiastic lecturer, much in demand both in the UK and abroad. In his obituary in the British Medical Journal, Bierer was remembered as one of the Jewish exiles from Austria and Nazi Germany who enriched British psychiatry and contributed widely to its present.[1]

As a person, Joshua Bierer was considered an upright man, caring, and full of humanity, and he fought for all those who were deprived and underprivileged. He was very proud of his Jewish heritage and with his twin brother, Immanuel, he co-founded the Movement of Hashomer Hatzair (the Young Guard) and two of the first kibbutzim in Israel (Beth Alpha and Mishmar HaEmek).[1]

Through the Institute of Social Psychiatry and the British Association of Social Psychiatry which he founded, Bierer was able to push forward community facilities for patients with longstanding and severe psychiatric disabilities. In this respect, he was a dedicated clinician. He founded and edited the *International Journal of Social Psychiatry* (in 1955) which he edited for many years and continued long after.[22]

A follower of Alfred Adler, he was strongly opposed to Freud's psychoanalytic theories and also the overuse of drugs in the treatment of mental illnesses. However, he did not consider himself as an antipsychiatrist and had reservations about the approach of RD Laing, his famous contemporary in London.[10] Bierer noted that schizophrenics needed treatment rather than the freedom to wallow in their delusions. His work was closer to that of Italian psychiatric reformer Franco Basaglia,[23] a leader in the

TABLE 1: Notable publications.

- The Day Hospital: An Experiment in Social Psychiatry and Syntho-analytic Psychotherapy (1951)
- Handbook of Community Psychiatry (1964, Bellak, Ed)
- (With RI Evans) Innovations in Social Psychiatry: A Social Psychological Perspective through Dialogue (1969)
- From Psychiatry to Social and Community Psychiatry (1980)

deinstitutionalization of mental health care. Noted patients of his included British writer Ian Fleming and painter Stanley Spencer.[24]

MAJOR CONTRIBUTIONS

These contributions are drawn from many sources: Bierer's books, abstracts of proceedings of his work, proceedings of lectures by him and other speakers, notes from Bierer's unpublished autobiography, "A Pedlar of Dreams" detailing his family background, his flight from Austria in the face of Nazism, and his approach to psychiatry, as well as the Runwell Hospital exhibition scrapbook (1939). The Wellcome Collection in London has an almost complete series of reprints by Bierer documenting his work (1948–1983), with news cuttings on the latter's clinical use of X-rays, file of draft letters to Margaret Thatcher and government health ministers and bodies, late 1970s to early 1980s, papers on the proposed closure of Marlborough Day Hospital, c.1980, news cuttings and photographs on Bierer's work and social psychiatry (1940s–1970s).[2,3]

The "Social" in Psychiatry

Bierer's contributions are broad and numerous. He is a pioneer, intellectual, and organizer. In addition to his pioneering work in psychiatry, Bierer was also very politically active. During his later years, he corresponded extensively with the British government, contributing advice on the reorganization of mental health care to the Principle Medical Officer of the National Health Service (NHS) and the Minister at the Department of Health and Social Security. An ardent admirer of Minister Margaret Thatcher, he wrote personally to the British Prime Minister.[2,3]

Newly cataloged material in The Wellcome Collection in London[2,3] relates particularly to the latter part of his career, includes extensive collections of news cuttings and photographs relating to his work and the operation of Marlborough Day Hospital. Of particular interest are drafts of his unpublished autobiography, "A Pedlar of Dreams," written toward the end of his life, which shed light on his varied life story and his approach to psychiatry. A few extracts will give a flavor of Bierer's concerns and commitments:

- "The psychiatric patient is a human being, the same as any of us. The psychiatric patient is no more the 'dangerous animal' one has to lock up."

- "All professionals working in the field of mental illness and maladjustment can be social psychiatrists."
- "'Mental illness' is an illness, a maladjustment, or a number of states and attitudes, or a combination of several factors. The psychiatric patient is not an object only, but an equal. We proved this by helping to open the doors of some mental hospitals."

Bierer's introduction of the principle of "self-determination" and "self-government" revolutionized the entire approach to mental illness and mental patients. Social psychiatry is not a school of thought but a movement, aiming at the mobilization of the democratic and human abilities and resources of the patient and the community in cooperation with a broadminded professional team, whose members have freed themselves of their prejudices against mental patients, using all modern methods of psychiatric and social prophylaxis, treatment, aftercare, and research, to achieve the best possible results in any case of an individual or group maladjustment or malfunction.[25]

Psychotherapy

Bierer's core work stems from a period in the 1940s and early 1950s when he tried to apply his insights as an Adlerian psychotherapist to general psychiatric practice. Bierer's work consistently emphasized the importance of the relationship between the individual and the social group. By applying these principles, he became a pioneer of group psychotherapy and the therapeutic community. He criticized the psychoanalytical theories of Freud and his followers, although he sought to distance himself from the antipsychiatry movement of thinkers such as RD Laing.[10] Bierer considered the day hospital as "part, or the forerunner, of an era which may be called tentatively the era of social psychiatry and syntho-analytic psychotherapy".[26]

As Norman Sartorius, Dinesh Bhugra, and other psychiatric leaders would later affirm,[27,28] Bierer held that all psychiatry was by its very nature "social," and that psychotherapy was analytic and synthetic in its techniques and objectives. Social psychiatry was defined by Bierer as the science that aims at the prevention and treatment of the suffering and poorly integrated individual or group in its universal setting, the latter implying all causes, including those of environment and relationship on the one hand, and constitution and physiology on the other. He incorporated Adlerian Therapy,[29] an encouragement-based counseling technique concentrating on prevention rather than mere remediation. It incorporated advising methods progressed to a combination of purposeful, psychodynamic views. It values the role of cooperation and connectedness among individuals in the world. Its ideology emphasizes the influence of personal choice, the fundamental nature of human beings, the significance of an idealistic and motivating life focus, the elimination of social inequality, and the prioritization of social relationships.

Social and Biological Components of Treatment

Bierer's approach to the treatment of mental illness was radical for its time and stood at odds with much of the international psychiatric community. He strongly opposed the overmedication of patients and emphasized the importance of rehabilitation and treatment in the community rather than in institutional settings.[30]

"I have just returned from the World Congress of Psychiatrists," he wrote. "There were hundreds of papers and discussions on the great value and success of the so-called medications. The whole Congress was one huge Drug Factory." In a telling case description, Bierer noted that, "after 1 month of intensive dynamic psychotherapy the patient threw all his drugs out of the window, he started to work, he became a 'HUMAN BEING'; and stopped being a 'chronic schizophrenic'".[30]

Hospital Treatments

The first psychiatric day hospitals in the Western World were opened simultaneously in 1946 by Bierer in London and Ewen Cameron in Montreal.[8] In an important paper, Bierer outlined the values and conceptual basis of his vision of a day hospital.[25] He believed that "mental patients should be met and treated in the same way as one meets and treats so-called normal people" and that "faulty or inadequate relationships are one of the causes of mental illness." Accordingly, "treatment of an experiential and situational nature, using the social group, is more effective." The description of the practice at the Marlborough Day Hospital is a fascinating mixture of the dated and the contemporary.[31] Diagnostic labels were avoided in favor of "as full a picture as possible of the total situation." Available treatments included "occupational therapy, individual psychotherapy or group therapy of a didactic, analytic, or psychoanalytic type, group discussions, social club therapy, art, drama, or physical treatment (such as electroconvulsive therapy, lysergic acid, insulin, tranquillizers, and abreaction)".[32] This heady mixture of social club, therapeutic community, and psychiatric clinic is apparent in many contemporary day hospitals and day centers. Whether this model of day care is appropriate to contemporary psychiatric practice was later questioned.[21]

Group Therapy and Community Treatments

Bierer's paper[33] reports an experiment with a new method of group therapy which combines: (1) Individual treatment; (2) group therapy; and (3) situational treatment. The experiment took the form of helping patients to run self-governed clubs, both in mental hospitals and in connection with the out-patient departments of voluntary hospitals. Conclusion: Not only are friendly relationships one function of human beings, but from a psychological point of view they are barometers of the state of health of each personality. A man without relationships not only feels the lack of them, but realizes that this lack is a sign of his failure in life. A lack of relationships is not the cause of mental illness, but merely a symptom. In curing that symptom, something much deeper is attacked. As the patient is assisted to make relationships, the proof of his failure is destroyed and a healthy personality begins to develop. It is comparatively easy for the psychotherapist to solve conflicts, but much more difficult to restore self-confidence. The problem of group psychotherapy is how to find a method which in a short time can produce good and lasting results, by a combination of analysis and re-education. The new approach just described aims at letting the patient himself experience situations which normally his deep conflicts prevent him from attempting. In this method, analysis follows rather than precedes the experience, and therefore the gulf between insight and realization is avoided.[33]

During 1 year's psychotherapeutic work at the Runwell Hospital for Nervous and Mental Diseases and in the Clinics of the Southend General and East Ham Memorial Hospitals, Bierer treated 70 neurotic and early psychotic patients with deep and intensive psychotherapy. Of these patients, 87% were cured or sufficiently improved to be discharged. In contrast to the Freudian method, the main features of Bierer's approach were: (1) Shortening of the time of analysis; (2) the combined usage of individual and group treatment; (3) the introduction of a method of situational treatment; (4) the introduction of new forms of social treatment; and (5) bridging the gulf which often exists between full insight and cure in psychoanalytical treatment.[33]

Psychopathic Behavior

Bierer also studied psychopathic behavior,[34] addressing the issue of psychopaths who have too much unlimited power. "With the advent of Nuclear Power, this danger has become a danger to the existence of this planet. It has become a most urgent task for the responsible people of this world to find a way to achieve a compulsory physical and mental examination of people with national and international power every 6 months. To say that it is impossible to achieve this is not good enough. Many things in History appeared impossible, but became possible 20–50 years later. The so-called 'Freedom of the Individual' which has been the most precious achievement of democracy should not be used to enable unscrupulous people to destroy this planet. Psychopathic behavior can be changed and new methods of treatment should be tried out. Dangerous psychopaths should be locked up, not in prisons, which is generally neither productive nor therapeutic. Where psychopaths could use their ambitions, their active brains in a constructive way, being useful to the community and to themselves and having been given the chance to go back to the community with enough savings in their hands and with the right advice how to use them. The limitation for the judges in

English Courts that psychiatric treatment can only be ordered for 1 year is sometimes useless. Judges should be given the right to order compulsory treatment for as long as therapeutically necessary or advisable. To enable us to think about and carry out these new experiments, it is essential that we change out ingrained opinion that psychopathic behavior cannot be changed."[34]

"Open-Door System"

In his paper on "Past, Present, and Future," Bierer[32] writes that "a great revolution—without doubt the greatest in history—is taking place in the field of mental health and mental illness." He advocates methods of the open-door system, community treatment, and both in- and out-patient departments in general hospitals.[31] The hospitals provide a day, night, and week-end shift; an out-patient department; child, parent, and marriage guidance, including a day ward for psychotic children; a therapeutic social club for each psychiatrist employed; a self-governed therapeutic community hostel; two community workshops; a community follow-up service; prophylactic services; and training facilities for psychiatrists, general practitioners, teachers, and paramedical workers. It concerns itself with the whole of the community and has an extended Community Service, indicating an open-door system.[31,35]

CURRENT STATUS

The "Social" in Psychiatry and Social Psychiatry

At the Fifth Joshua Bierer Memorial Lecture delivered to the British Association for Social Psychiatry in 1991, RH Cawley stated that: "From my audacious method of judging the present day value of precepts which were set out 40 years ago, Bierer's six principles of social psychiatry have not done too badly".[36] The six principles are—"universality, relatedness, conation, centripetal-centrifugal interaction, multidimensional approach, and experiential treatment" which were cogent in their time and context also applicable to today's interventions.

In the 1993 Bierer Memorial Lecture, Sheldon[24] explores how research on the interrelationship between biological, social, and psychological factors in mental disorders has been reflected in changes to the services available to patients and caregivers. Ideology and irrationality, biological, psychological, and social dimensions of mental disorders, such as social isolation, low SES, and unemployment in mental disorder are noted. Several other studies highlight the psychosocial determinants that contribute to causation, maintenance, and recovery from symptoms and suffering and enhance positives.[24] The WHO Commission called on all governments to lead global action on the social determinants of health with the aim of achieving health equity.[13,37]

Psychiatric Treatment

Bierer's papers incorporate many of the practices that he preached and practiced in psychiatric treatments. Psychiatry and society are interrelated and the biopsychosocial model continues to dominate the clinical psychiatric practice. Advances in neurosciences, neurobiology, and genetics tend to swing the emphasis toward a more biological basis. Yet, the symptoms of hallucinations and delusions in psychosis have social meaning for the person experiencing them and are primarily defined socially. The vulnerability is often the result of social trauma, whether in the form of recent stressors that trigger onset, or earlier circumstances that shape cognitive and emotional style. The approved treatment and management of long-term psychiatric disorders has involved interventions that are either directly social, or psychosocial. Although psychiatric disorders have been approached primarily from a biological perspective, social factors still have an important role in cross-cultural diagnosis, psychiatric disorders relating to social deprivation, rehabilitation, and enabling social inclusion.

Psychiatrist and medical anthologists Arthur Kleinman and associates[38] argue that narrowing research to biological research approaches is of decreasing relevance to clinical practice and global health, and should include greater support for researchers conducting social, clinical, and community studies within a broad, more humanistic biosocial framework. Kingsley Norton[39] identified five key therapeutic functions of the ward environment (containment, support, structure, involvement, and validation) and four destructive processes related to the isolated patient, group phenomena, the contribution of staff, and structural manifestations in the ward. The inpatient ward can be construed as a "whole," embodying a range of therapeutic functions, which may need rapid deployment and dismantling, as dictated by changes in ward conditions. He recommends a "ward-as-a-whole" construct complements of individualized models of patient care and the practical implications of such thinking could engender a greater sense of agency and job satisfaction in staff.

Psychotherapies

"In no other branch of medicine have doctors appeared so nihilistic or so defeatist as in the domain of psychiatry," Bierer[26] declared. "It seems to me questionable whether this is due to the disparity in the therapeutic results between psychiatry on the one hand and general medicine on the other. In general medicine, it is frequently forgotten that the really specific remedies at our disposal are so few that they can be counted on the fingers of one hand. If, on the other hand, we remember that as late as the time of the French Revolution mental patients were kept in chains, and that to-day in modem hospitals we see impressive results with such specific treatments as malarial therapy, then it must be admitted that the psychiatrist is not the only nihilist;

but that this also applies to representatives of other branches of general medicine. If, however, the psychiatrist appears to be the greater nihilist, this is, in my opinion, due to the fact that in each of us there is the unconscious conviction that in our relationship with our patients, behind our hypodermic syringe lies something else, something personal and individual, which we believe we are unable to grasp. It is now nearly half a century since Freud published his first book. There is no doubt that his productions, like those of Adler, Jung, Meyer, etc., have caused a revolution; or at least have profoundly influenced scientific thought. How much, however, have they influenced the nihilism of the psychiatrist? I am afraid not much. No doubt they have on the one hand contributed a great deal to our understanding of mental patients; but on the other hand they have stimulated false hopes of cure which often were transformed into bitter disappointments."

Although Bierer was a grateful pupil of Adler and appreciated the genius of Freud, he held that, "We shall need to find the simplest and most natural expression for our theoretical doctrines. It would be difficult to do so, as a scientific foundation of psychotherapy as a natural science would have to be based on experiment. It is not gratifying that the results vary from 26 to 88%. On the other hand, one reads papers that show normal remission rates with occupational therapy or with prolonged narcosis up to 46%. It is a good thing that we sometimes forget that we cannot prove the direct efficiency of our treatment, and that many cases recover not because of, but in spite of, our help." As Bleuler sarcastically points out, treating "pneumonia takes twenty-one days with the aid of a good physician, three weeks without his aid; and with the aid of a bad physician much longer. Is psychiatry really in such a bad plight? I think not. It is true we cannot offer a scientific foundation, and we prefer not to rely upon an apparent one. Up to now, unfortunately, the only measure we have is that of result".[26]

CONCLUDING REMARKS

Dr Salman Akhtar, who contributed the chapter on Karen Horney to this volume, recounts a telling anecdote about Joseph Bierer that gives us the measure of the man: "I met Joshua Bierer in the mid-70s when I was a resident in the department of psychiatry at UVA School of Medicine in Charlottesville, VA. John Beckman MD, our residency director and a Polish-British immigrant to USA, had had a deep relationship with Bierer during his years in the UK. He invited Bierer to our department for a week long teaching stint."

During his visit to UVA, Bierer "emphasized the importance of group processes and of the societal surround upon the development and functioning of an individual." "More importantly," Akhtar concludes, "I was impressed by his iconoclastic, larger than life, Lear-like persona. He took to me kindly and over the next few years published three or four papers of mine in the journal he had founded in 1955, *The International Journal of Social Psychiatry*."

Joshua Bierer founded the International Association for Social Psychiatry (IASP), which became WASP as of the 2nd Congress of Social Psychiatry that also took place in London, UK. As the successor to the IASP, WASP is now in its 60th year which will celebrated at the 25th World congress of Social Psychiatry in Marrakech, Morocco in 2026. The movement Bierer started is thriving through WASP and 27 national associations and several affiliated groups from Argentina and The Philippines to the West African group forming a fledgling association.[6] WASP has published a textbook of social psychiatry[40] and publishes a new journal, *World Social Psychiatry* founded in 2019, that continues in the spirit of Joshua Bierer.

Since social conditions change, each generation has to redefine the meaning of social psychiatry, its relevance, and its application to its own social conditions—and not only globally but locally.[4,37] To take social psychiatry seriously is to take social conditions and social changes seriously and that is why today's social psychiatry must be updated from Joshua Bierer's social psychiatry and why social psychiatry in Canada is different from its North American neighbor, the USA, and both are very different than the associations in South America like Brazil, and India and Japan in Asia, to name a few examples.

Bierer was a catalyst for many health and social services trends in the postwar world in Europe and North America, where we saw a humanistic movement from institutions to the community, with a growing appreciation of the impacts of social class,[11,12] social stress,[17] adverse childhood experiences,[14] and the Social Determinants of Health,[13] all in the light of serious sociological[19] and philosophical critiques[41] of psychiatry of the 1960s. As an innovator and a pioneer, Bierer was an expansive advocate for the cause of deinstitutionalizing mental illness,[42] taking the broadest view of social psychiatry in practice,[43] and presciently anticipating what we now call the Social Determinants of Health and Mental Health.[13,44] His influence was powerful, along with that of others, in shifting the climate of opinion about the social dimensions of mental illness to create a more compassionate and humanistic approach to its treatment.[4,30]

REFERENCES

1. Obituary: Joshua Bierer. Br Med J. 1985;ccxc:163.
2. Wellcome Collection. Bierer, Dr Joshua. [online] Available from https://wellcomecollection.org/search/works?query=joshua+bierer. [Last accessed February, 2025]
3. Consortium for History of Science, Medicine and Technology. Wellcome Collection Makes Papers of Dr. Joshua Bierer Available for Research. [online] Available from https://www.chstm.org/news/wellcome-collection-makes-papers-dr-joshua-bierer-available-research. [Last accessed February 2025].
4. Di Nicola V. "A person is a person through other persons": A manifesto for 21st century social psychiatry. In: Gogineni RR, Pumariega AJ, Kallivayalil R,

Kastrup M, Rothe EM (Eds). The WASP Textbook on Social Psychiatry: Historical, Developmental, Cultural, and Clinical Perspectives. New York, NY: Oxford University Press; 2023. pp. 44-67.

5. Ferreira AG. The life of WASP from 1964 to 1992. [online] Available from https://waspsocialpsychiatry.org/history/. [Last accessed February, 2025]
6. Kallivayalil RA, Kastrup M, Gogineni RR, Di Nicola V, Sharma S. History of social psychiatry and historical aspects of the World Association of Social Psychiatry. In: Gogineni RR, Pumariega AJ, Kallivayalil R, Kastrup M, Rothe EM (Eds). The WASP Textbook on Social Psychiatry: Historical, Developmental, Cultural, and Clinical Perspectives. New York, NY: Oxford University Press; 2023. pp. 9-22.
7. Lyons A. Psychiatric Day Hospitals. Ulster Med J. 2020;89(1):34-7.
8. Goldman DL. Two pioneers of today's partial hospital and their ideas. Int J Partial Hosp. 1990;6(2):181-8.
9. Di Nicola V. Special Communication—Attachment, Family, and Social Systems: London's "Cradle to Grave" Contributions as a Model for Social Psychiatry. World Soc Psychiatry. 2023;5(1):21-8.
10. Laing RD, Esterson A. Sanity, Madness and the Family. London: Penguin Books; 1964.
11. Young M, Willmott P. Family and Kinship in East London. London: Routledge & Kegan Paul; 1957.
12. Sennett R, Cobb J. The Hidden Injuries of Class. London, UK: Verso; 2023.
13. CSDH. Closing the Gap in a Generation: Health Equity through Action on the Social Determinants of Health Final Report of the Commission on Social Determinants of Health. Geneva: World Health Organization; 2008.
14. Felitti VJ, Anda RF. The relationship of adverse childhood experiences to adult medical disease, psychiatric disorders and sexual behavior: implications for health care. In: Lanius RA, Vermette E, Pain C (Eds). The Impact of Early Trauma on Health and Disease: The Hidden Epidemic. Cambridge, UK: Cambridge University Press; 2010. pp. 77-87.
15. Gunderson JG, Will OA, Mosher LR. Principles and Practice of Milieu Therapy. New York, NY: Jason Aronson; 1983.
16. Jones M. Social Psychiatry in Practice: The Idea of the Therapeutic Community Harmondsworth, UK: Penguin; 1968.
17. Rosen G. Social stress and mental disease from the eighteenth century to the present: Some origins of social psychiatry. Millbank Mem Fund Q. 1959;37(1):5-32.
18. Frank LK. Society as the patient. Am J Sociol. 1936;42:335-44.
19. Goffman E. Asylums: Essays on the Social Situation of Mental Patients and Other Inmates. New York, NY: Anchor Books; 1961.
20. Smith M. The First Resort: The History of Social Psychiatry in the United States. New York, NY: Columbia University Press; 2023.
21. Holloway F. Joshua Bierer and social psychiatry. Int J Soc Psychiatry. 1992;38(2):85-6.
22. Fuzeki V. Bierer and social psychiatry. Int J Soc Psychiatry. 1979;25(4):240-2.
23. Basaglia F, Scheper-Hughes N, Lovell AM. Psychiatry Inside Out: Selected Writings of Franco Basaglia. New York, NY: Columbia University Press; 1987.
24. Sheldon B. The social and biological components of mental disorder: Implications for services: The 1993 Joshua Bierer Memorial Lecture. Int J Soc Psychiatry. 1994;4(2):87-105.

25. Bierer J. The Therapeutic Community Hostel. Int J Soc Psychiatry. 1960;7(1):5-10.
26. Bierer J. Psychotherapy in mental hospital practice. J Ment Sci. 1940; 86(364):928-52.
27. Sartorius N, Gaebel W, López-Ibor JJ, Maj M. Psychiatry in Society. Chichester, UK: John Wiley and Sons; 2002. p. 27.
28. Ventriglio A, Gupta S, Bhugra D. Why do we need a social psychiatry? Br J Psychiatry. 2016;209:1-2.
29. Cedeno R, Torrico TJ. (2024). Adlerian Therapy. [online] Available from https://www.ncbi.nlm.nih.gov/books/NBK599518/. [Last accessed February, 2025]
30. Bierer J. Crisis in Medicine (Humanity). Int J Soc Psychiatry. 1980;26(1):5-6.
31. Bierer J. The Day Hospital: An Experiment in Social Psychiatry and Synthoanalytic Psychotherapy. London, UK: H. K. Lewis; 1951.
32. Bierer J. Past, Present and Future. Int J Soc Psychiatry. 1960;6(3-4):165-73.
33. Bierer J, Lieut RAMC. A New Form of Group Psychotherapy. Ment Health (Lond). 1944;5(2):23-6.
34. Bierer J. Can Psychopathic Behaviour Be Changed? Int J Soc Psychiatry. 1977;23(4):291-303.
35. Bierer J, Haldane FP. A self-governed patients' social club in a public mental hospital. J Ment Sci. 1941;87(368):419-26.
36. Cawley RH. Bierer's Precepts Today and Tomorrow: The Fifth Joshua Bierer Memorial Lecture delivered to the British Association for Social Psychiatry, 23 May 1991. Int J Soc Psychiatry. 1992;38(2):87-94.
37. Di Nicola V. Review article—The Global South: an emergent epistemology for social psychiatry. World Soc Psychiatry. 2020;2(1):20-6.
38. Kleinman A, Eisenberg L, Good B. Culture, illness, and care: clinical lessons from anthropologic and cross-cultural research. Ann Intern Med. 1978;88(2):251-8.
39. Norton K. Re-thinking acute psychiatric inpatient care. Int J Soc Psychiatry. 2004;50(3):274-84.
40. Gogineni RR, Pumariega AJ, Kallivayalil RA, Kastrup M, Rothe EM. The WASP Textbook on Social Psychiatry: Historical, Developmental, Cultural, and Clinical Perspectives. New York, NY: Oxford University Press; 2023.
41. Foucault M. Madness and Civilization: A History of Insanity in the Age of Reason. New York, NY: Vintage; 1973.
42. Bierer J. From psychiatry to social and community psychiatry. Int J Soc Psychiatry. 1980;26(2):77-9.
43. Bierer J, Evans RI. Innovations in Social Psychiatry: A Social Psychological Perspective Through Dialogue. London, UK: Avenue Publishing Co.; 1969.
44. Bierer J. What social psychiatry means to me! Int J Soc Psychiatry. 1973;19(1-2):1-3.

George Morrison Carstairs

Mohan Isaac

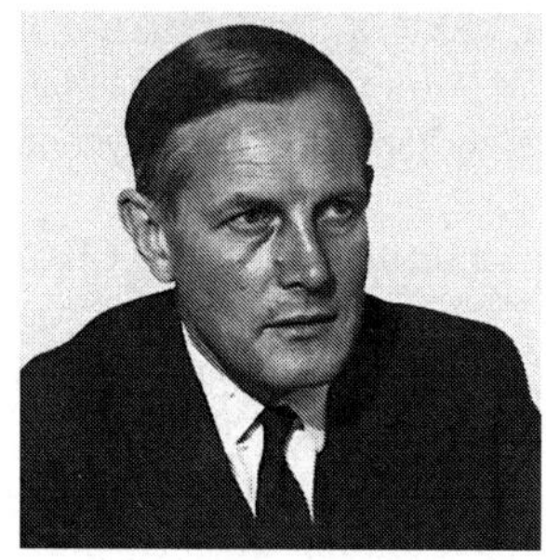

(1916–1991)

INTRODUCTION

The 1950s and 1960s were a time of rapid and radical transformation in the field of mental health care and services in Britain and all over the western, developing world. Growing concerns about the welfare of persons with mental disorders during the previous 50–100 years, contributed to the growth of moral and humane treatment in public mental asylums which were built in ideal locations in most industrialized countries. The mental asylums steadily grew in numbers as also the number of inpatients in such asylums. The second half of the 19th century and the early part of the first half of 20th century can be referred to as the period of "rise of the asylums". But conditions in the asylums began to decline from the beginning of the 20th century due to various reasons such as ever-increasing number of admissions, serious overcrowding, poorer sanitary and living conditions, and dwindling financial support (during the war time and later). Social situation of patients and inmates of asylums and ill effects of long-term stay in asylums were systematically studied by few sociologists and psychiatrists notably Erving Goffman who wrote about the characteristics of total institutions,[1] Russell Barton who described the features of "institutional neurosis",[2] George Brown and John Wing who talked about the development of secondary handicaps[3] and Ernest Gruenberg who identified the "social breakdown syndrome".[4] The growing professional and public perception that asylums were not healthy and therapeutic institutions but perhaps harmful places for persons with mental disorders initiated a period of the "fall of asylums" which ultimately began with the serendipitous discovery of the first pharmacological agent to treat the mentally ill, chlorpromazine, during the early 1950s. Psychiatrists were becoming increasingly accepting of the negative effects of the hospital environment on the mental health of patients. The deinstitutionalization movement had begun with widespread use of chlorpromazine, discharging of large number of patients from asylums into the community and closing of either part or the whole of the asylum.

During the 1950s and 1960s, there was also steady growth of interest in social and cultural influences on the genesis and evolution of mental ill health and the community prevalence of mental disorders. Several major studies such as the ecological study of mental disorders by Faris and Dunham (1939) in Chicago,[5] the mid-town Manhattan study by Leo Srole et al. (1962)[6] and the Stirling County study by Leighton et al. (1963)[7] were initiated and completed during this period. It was during this tumultuous period, early days of community care of the mentally ill in Britain and elsewhere that George Morrison (Morris) Carstairs decided to specialize in psychiatry. Much of Morris Carstairs' major contributions to social and community psychiatry and development of mental health care in less developed countries were made during the 1950s to 1970s period.

BRIEF BIOGRAPHY

George Morrison Carstairs (Morris) was born on 18th June, 1916 in Mussoorie, a hill station near Dehradun City, on the foothills of the Himalayas (about 290 kilometers away from Delhi, the national capital of India) in British India (British Raj). Mussoorie is in the present Indian state of Uttarakhand. His father, Reverend Dr George Carstairs, was a distinguished and dedicated Church of Scotland minister and missionary working in British India with the Rajputana (present day Rajasthan state in India) Mission and his mother was Elizabeth Hurley Young. Morris's paternal grandfather, Reverend George Lindley Carstairs, too was an ordained minister. Morris spent his formative childhood period, the first 9 years of his life, growing up in Mussoorie when he learnt and became fluent in Hindi. As he grew up, Morris began to share his father's passion for India which stayed with him all his life. In some of his later writings, he has written about his fond memories of "playing marbles and other local games with a pack of little Hindu boys" and "touring the countryside by bullock carts". He and his family moved to Edinburgh, Scotland when he was 10 years. Morris completed his schooling at George Watson's College, then a private, all-boys school in Edinburgh. This dramatic shift in cultural ecology perhaps laid the foundation of Morris's later interest in the impact of sociocultural variables in mental life.

During his late teens and early 20s, Morris was an accomplished long-distance runner who participated and won prizes in athletics championships.

He was the Scottish 3 miles champion in 1937, 1938, and 1939. He cloaked championship best of 14 minutes and 35.8 seconds in 1937.[8] He represented Scotland and Great Britain in the European Athletics Championships of 1938, coming sixth in the 5,000 meters with a time of 14:51.3. He also won the silver medal in the 5,000 meters at the World Students Games of 1937 and the gold in 1939.

Morris decided to study medicine and joined the University of Edinburgh. At the university, he read arts as well as medicine at the medical school. He was a medalist in Fine Art[9] and he graduated Bachelor of Medicine and Bachelor of Surgery (MBChB) in 1941. Following his graduation, he joined the Royal Edinburgh Hospital as an assistant physician in general medicine.[10] The Second World War was on then and in 1942, Morris was called up for active war service as a medical officer. He was commissioned (emergency commission) into the medical branch of the Royal Air Force Volunteer Service as a Flying Officer. After a year of service in the medical branch, he was promoted to the next higher rank of Flight Lieutenant. He served in Europe and the Far East. After the war ended, he was demobilized from service in 1946.

While serving as medical officer during the war, Morris became interested in social anthropology, particularly in studies of the influence of cultural environments in personality development.[9] So, he studied social anthropology both at Cambridge and in the USA under leading anthropologists namely Sir Evans-Pritchard, Meyer Fortes, and Alexander Leighton. He held research fellowship for the next couple of years to further study anthropology and carry out anthropological field work and research. He went to New York as a Commonwealth Fund Fellow during 1948–1949 when he received training in culture and personality approach to psychological anthropology under Margaret Mead in preparation for field studies.[10] During 1949–1951, he carried out anthropological field work living in primitive village communities in Rajasthan, India. During part of this time, Morris held a Rockefeller grant and a fellowship from the Henderson Trust. His research in Rajasthan is published in his book "The Twice Born."

Morris married Vera Hunt, a graduate in economics, sociology, and statistics from the University College London and London School of Economics (LSE) in December 1950. Vera joined him in Rajasthan, India in 1951 to assist him in field research which contributed to his book "The Twice Born".[11] Vera later joined the Scotland civil service as a social researcher and statistician. During the several years of her services for the Scottish Home and Health Department in various capacities, Vera made significant contributions including the "Carstairs Index of Deprivation".[11] Morris and Vera had three children—two sons and a daughter.

In 1953, Morris was appointed as a Senior Registrar in psychiatry at the Maudsley Hospital in London where he worked with chronic psychiatric

TABLE 1: Notable publications.

- This Island Now (The B.B.C. Reith Lecture 1962) (1963)
- CARSTAIRS GM. This island now. Br Med J. 1963 Jan 19;1(5324):141-6. doi: 10.1136/bmj.1.5324.141. PMID: 14018929; PMCID: PMC2123348.
- *The Twice-Born:* A Study of A Community of High-caste Hindus (1957)
- Adrian C. Mayer, The Twice-Born: A Study of a Community of High-Caste Hindus, International Affairs, Volume 34, Issue 3, July 1958, Page 398, https://doi.org/10.2307/2605248
- *Death of a Witch:* A Village in North India, 1950–1981 (1983)
- Carstairs, G. M. (1974). *Death of a witch: A village in North India 1950-1981*. Hutchinson.
- *The Great Universe of Kota:* Stress, Change, and Mental Disorder in an Indian Village (1976)
- Psychiatric Problems of Developing Countries. British Journal of Psychiatry. 123:271-77 (1973)

patients, under the supervision and guidance of Sir Aubrey Lewis, the first Professor of Psychiatry at the Institute of Psychiatry and Maudsley Hospital. Morris also joined the Medical Research Council (MRC) Social Psychiatry Unit under Sir Aubrey. Based on his studies of the chronic mentally ill, discharged from the hospital, Morris wrote his research thesis on "Chronic mental illness: a study of clinical and social factors related to the outcome of patients discharged from mental hospitals" and obtained his MD degree from the University of Edinburgh in 1959. In 1960, he was appointed Director of a new Medical Research Council Unit for Epidemiological Studies in Psychiatry in London. In the very next year, in 1961, Morris was appointed to the Chair of Psychological Medicine at the University of Edinburgh as Professor. Edinburgh's medical school was one of the first in the English-speaking world to offer specialized teaching on mental disorders. It was also the first school to create a chair of psychiatry.[12] When he moved to Edinburgh, the MRC psychiatric epidemiology unit moved with him. Morris was elected a member of the Harveian Society of Edinburgh in 1962. He continued as Professor and Chair at Edinburgh until 1973 when he was appointed the second Vice Chancellor of York University. While at Edinburgh, Morris was elected the President of the World Federation of Mental Health from 1968 to 1972. During this period and later, he also assisted the World Health Organization (WHO) in various capacities. After 5 years as Vice Chancellor of York University, Morris relinquished the post in 1978 and moved to India where he was a Visiting Professor of Psychiatry at three leading institutes namely the National Institute of Mental Health and Neurosciences (NIMHANS) in Bangalore, Postgraduate Institute of Medical Education and Research (PGIMER) in Chandigarh, and the All India Institute of Medical Sciences (AIIMS) in New Delhi. He completed his ongoing anthropological observations and studies in villages in Rajasthan during this 3-year period.

The writing of the work was subsequently completed (which resulted in his final book, "Death of a Witch") in the United States where Morris was a Fellow of the Woodrow Wilson Center in Washington, DC.

Morris developed progressive cognitive decline (dementia) in his later years and had to withdraw from academia and professional life. He died at his Edinburgh home on 17th April 1991.

MAJOR CONTRIBUTIONS

It was during 1955–1956 that the use of the newly discovered tranquilizing medication, chlorpromazine, became widespread in industrialized countries such as the USA and Britain. Morris had begun his academic work at the MRC Social Psychiatry Unit at the Maudsley in 1953. His initial academic and research interest was the chronic mentally ill patient incarcerated for years inside the mental hospital, who now had an opportunity to get discharged into the community and home. While taking over as the Chair of Psychiatry at Edinburgh, in his inaugural lecture, in 1961, Morris declared that his particular interest which he hoped to pursue as chair was social psychiatry.[12] He said that his desire was to follow in the footsteps of two leading British psychiatrists of his time, Sir David Henderson (former chair of psychiatry in Edinburgh), and Sir Aubrey Lewis both of whom believed mental illnesses to be a social and public health problem requiring also involvement of general practitioners and primary care medical officers. They also believed in the role of and need for preventive action. During those early days of the deinstitutionalization movement, Morris's contributions were in social and community psychiatry. Like his mentors, Morris too believed in the importance of social and cultural influences in the genesis and maintenance of mental disorders. His love of India made him contribute significantly to the development of mental health services in developing countries such as India.[13] His contributions to the developing countries were facilitated by his long association with the Department of Mental Health of the WHO and World Federation of Mental Health. Besides being a clinician and researcher, Morris was an avid teacher and role model. He believed in appropriate training in psychiatry for all medical students and in establishing standards for postgraduate training in psychiatry. His major contributions could be considered under the following areas: (1) Social and community psychiatry, (2) psychiatry education both at the graduate and postgraduate levels, (3) psychiatric epidemiology, (4) commentary on the British society, (5) social anthropological study of Hindu character in India, and (6) psychiatry in developing countries.

Social and Community Psychiatry

By the mid-1950s, the structure and functions as well as the numbers and composition of admissions of mental hospitals were beginning to change. One of Morris's earlier studies was a census of all patients of four mental hospitals in London area (on July 12, 1954).[14] The study showed that hospital records, census, and statistics (patients demographic background, age, occupation, social class, diagnosis at the time of admission, and length of stay) were inadequate for an epidemiological understanding of mental disorders. More sophisticated methods of data collection from the community are needed.

Another study in the mid-1950s showed that organization of an industrial workshop inside the mental hospital, in which mental hospital patients were paid for their work, can be effectively used as an instrument for rehabilitation of chronic mental patients. It also showed that many long-stay patients can reach normal levels of rate of work at comparatively unskilled tasks.[15,16] The study highlighted the importance of the concept that regular and useful work can play a role in preventing deterioration of long-stay patients. Regular attendance at the workshop was associated in many cases with appreciable improvement in patients' social behavior. An accessory social influence namely the attitude of staff toward the patient was also important for improved social behavior.[17]

Although increasing number of chronic and long-stay patients were discharged into the community, the level at which they were functioning, their post-hospital adjustment, problems faced by their families in managing them, and clinical and social factors related to their outcome were not known. Most such patients had varying degrees of residual disability. Outcome of 227 of the 240 patients discharged from 7 mental hospitals in and around London between July 1949 and June 1956 were studied.[18] Successful outcome was associated with patients' clinical state on discharge and with their subsequent employment. Patients being employed also made it easier for their family members to manage them. It was also noticed that many patients who were unemployed were judged to be capable of working and could have benefitted from "sheltered employment". Patients staying with siblings or in lodgings had better outcome in terms of relapse or rehospitalization than those staying with parents, with wives, or in large hostels. The need of discharged patients and their families for continued and supportive social work was highlighted.

The influence of family life on the course of schizophrenic illness was studied by Morris and his colleagues at the MRC Social Psychiatry Unit.[19] An elegant and methodologically sophisticated 1 year follow-up study using standardized assessment instruments of 128 males with schizophrenia who were discharged from mental hospitals showed that 55% deteriorated during the first year after discharge, three quarters of these patients were readmitted at least once during the year. The study revealed that patients who returned to a relative who showed "high emotional involvement" (based on measures of expressed emotion, hostility, and dominance) deteriorated more frequently than patients who returned to a relative who showed "low emotional involvement".[20]

The second half of the 1950s was a time when psychiatric outpatient clinics were opening in general hospitals and attendances at such clinics were steadily increasing. Morris carried out sociological observations of psychiatric outpatient clinics in Britain and studied one psychiatric outpatient clinic in the USA (New-Haven, Connecticut).[21] It was observed that the norm of treatment offered in outpatient clinics was different in Britain and in the USA. In the former, short-term treatments with relatively brief interviews and much reliance on drug therapy was the rule; in the latter relatively long-term treatment, with an emphasis on extensive psychotherapeutic interviews, was the preferred approach.

Psychiatric Education Both at the Graduate and Postgraduate Levels

All his life, Morris was recognized as a great teacher, mentor, guide, and role model. While he was the Chair of Psychological Medicine at Edinburgh from 1961 to 1973, he was able to gather round him some distinguished colleagues and a galaxy of bright students who later became eminent themselves. He built the department into a center of international reputation known for excellence in research, undergraduate and postgraduate psychiatric education, and clinical practice. Morris served as a member of the Royal Commission on Medical Education which was set up in 1965 to review medical education, undergraduate and postgraduate, in Great Britain.[22] A survey of undergraduate psychiatric teaching in the United Kingdom conducted by Morris and his colleagues showed that there was great diversity in the amount, content, and methods of teaching psychiatry in the UK medical schools. No two schools were quite alike in the type of staff facilities, in the allocation of teaching time in the several years of the course, or in the persons available to act as teachers.[23] As a member of the Royal Commission on Medical Education, Morris was able to highlight the significance of integrating adequate and appropriate training in psychiatry in a uniform manner in all medical schools.

As the demand for psychiatric care was becoming evident all over the world, the need for trained psychiatrists even in rich, developed countries was increasingly realized. In 1963, Morris assisted the Expert Committee on Mental Health of the WHO to deliberate on and make recommendations about training of psychiatrists.[24] The committee reviewed the need for psychiatrists and the availability of psychiatrists as well as psychiatric training across the world. It examined in detail of the background requirements for specialization in psychiatry, the patterns, methods and organization of training, and the role of WHO in training of psychiatrists. Of the 109 countries reviewed, wide variations were found in the number of psychiatrists per 100,000 population available. The numbers ranged from 0 for 8 countries (with a combined population of about 20 million) to >7 per 100,000 in one country. Most countries had only up to 0.49 and only 8 countries had over 4. The percentage of psychiatrists employed in public institutions differed greatly. Standards of psychiatry training, both the intensity and quality, were very different across the countries. Morris contributed in various ways to develop and improve psychiatric training in various parts of the world but most importantly in developing countries.

Epidemiology of Psychiatric Disorders

Morris's interest in psychiatric epidemiology blossomed while he began work at the MRC Social Psychiatry Unit in London where he conducted a hospital statistics-based study in mental hospitals.[13] He was appointed the first director of the newly created MRC Unit for Epidemiological Studies in Psychiatry in London in 1960. The Unit moved with him when he took over as the chair in Edinburgh. Morris carried out a survey of psychiatric morbidity in two communities, a mining, and an agricultural community in South Wales.[25] A count was made of psychiatric cases, attempted suicides, suicides, and crimes of violence occurring during a five- and half-year period in these two defined communities. Cases occurred at the rate 3.8 per 1,000 of population aged over 15 years per annum in the mining valley and 2.6 per 1,000 per annum in the agricultural area. In the mining valley, suicides were twice as frequent among men; in the agricultural area women outnumbered men in all categories except suicide. This study was an attempt to relate the prevalence of psychiatric disorders in two communities to sociological differences between the populations at risk and establish the degree to which socioenvironmental factors contribute to the recognition and management of mental illness.

As the Chair of Psychological Medicine at Edinburgh University and Director of the MRC Unit for Epidemiological Studies in Psychiatry, Morris believed in the application of epidemiological principles to social psychiatry and combining epidemiology with clinical studies. His department and unit were well known for authoritatively studying the social and psychological concomitants of attempted suicides. Until the momentous decision to decriminalize suicides in 1961, attempted suicide was a punishable offence in England and Wales. But, from 1961, attempted suicides were treated as a medical and social problem and all cases of attempted suicides brought to a hospital were assessed by a psychiatrist. Deliberate self-poisoning most commonly overdosing with barbiturate hypnotics were becoming more and more common and a matter of public concern.[26,27] Morris himself has written about the characteristics of the Suicide-Prone, highlighting that the warning of a suicidal gesture, and even of expressed suicidal intent, must never pass unheeded.[28] He prescribed several tasks and some targets for future epidemiological research in psychiatry.[29]

Years later, during the early 1970s, Morris, in collaboration with one of his former doctoral students at Edinburgh and an Indian psychiatrist, Ravinder Lal Kapur carried out a major survey of the prevalence and patterns of mental disorders in a rural setting in India—in Kota, a village in the southwest cost of India, in South Kanara district of Karnataka state of India, among three caste groups namely brahmins (priestly class), bunts (agriculturists), and mogers (local fishermen).[30] They studied stress and social change in these communities as some of them were moving from a matrilineal to a patrilineal system of inheritance. The results of this survey published as a book—"The Great Universe of Kota: Stress, Change, and Mental Disorders in an Indian Village" is considered as an important contribution to psychiatric epidemiology in India.

Commentary on the British Society

Morris was chosen to deliver the prestigious BBC (British Broadcasting Corporation) Reith Lectures in 1962—BBC's flagship annual lecture series delivered by significant international thinkers, broadcast on BBC radio to a global audience via the BBC's Overseas and Transcription Services. The Reith Lectures, named in honor of the first director general of the BBC, Sir John Reith, to mark his contribution to the idea of public service broadcasting, allowed a speaker to talk at length on a subject in the "field of thought". In a series of six lectures titled "the island now" [which included (1) the stability and change in social environment, (2) the first years, (3) vicissitudes of adolescence, (4) the changing role of women, (5) living and partly living, and (6) the changing British character], Morris described various aspects of the then British society and the effects of the social environment on the mental health of individuals.[31,32] He explored the lifestyle of the Britons, gave his scholarly analysis of the society, and touched upon numerous issues such as growth and development of children, national patterns and problems of teenagers, the adolescent crisis, rules governing sexual behavior, sex, and violence, increase of crimes, changing role of women, psychological consequences of social change, the decay of faith ("loss of conviction in any suprapersonal system of values") and causes of sickness in the then British society. The transcripts and audio recordings of all the six lectures can be freely downloaded from "BBC Radio 4 - The Reith Lectures" (https://www.bbc.co.uk/programmes/b00729d9).

In his Reith lectures, Morris also suggested solutions for malaise of the society. He said, "I believe that it is time that our society awakened to the need for clearer self-knowledge as a means to remedying some of the current disorders in our private and public life" "I suggest that the ultimate value behind attempts to remedy the diverse patterns of social failure is simply this: a belief in the individual worth and dignity, of every human being".[31] Some of his observations, for example his condoning of premarital sex ("premarital sexual exploration might be healthy for relationships") became very controversial. He cautioned about the promise of and the high hopes on the benefits of the newly discovered medications for all kinds of mental disorders and said "to relieve emotional stress which is caused by problems of living, they are merely an anodyne. To ally the symptoms while failing to explore and if possible, eradicate, the cause has always been bad medicine".[32]

Social Anthropological Study of Hindu Character in India

Morris always talked about his allegiance to two cultures—"to the ancient society of India" in which he spent his early years and to "the middle-aged society of Britain." He devoted 2 years of field work in social anthropology living in a village near Udaipur in Rajasthan, India during the early 1950s studying the Hindu personality structure. He studied members of three higher Indian castes—the "twice born" casts, the Rajputs (warriors and landlords), Brahmins (priests), and Banias (merchants). 37 male informants, 11 Brahmins, 13 Rajputs, and 13 Banias were interviewed at length in a nondirective manner to study the Hindu upper caste male social character. Morris wanted to explore the part played by early formative experiences in determining adult personality and see how certain psychological characteristics of a community were reflected in the personalities of its individual members. The results of the study published as a book titled "The Twice-Born"[33] which had a preface by Margaret Mead was widely reviewed and credited as a study on Hinduism and national character.

The study contributed to understanding of the sexual life of individuals of these upper castes, how religious beliefs influenced relationship between men and women and attitudes toward homosexuality.[34] The widespread hypochondriac concern over "jiryan" or spermatorrhea was considered as the most common expression of anxiety neurosis among the communities in rural areas of Rajasthan.[34]

During the field work, living for nearly 2 years in villages of Rajasthan in northwestern India, Morris conducted a regular medical clinic. He notes that to effectively function as a doctor in an Indian village, one must understand various Indian concepts of disease causation and management such as the concept of "bodily heat and cold," role of different kind of food stuff, the role of religion and faith, the need for rituals, prayers, and pilgrimages as components of treatment, belief in ghosts, evil spirits, possession, black magic, and the significant role of faith healers and other traditional healers.[35]

Based on his encounters with death and suicides during his medical work in the villages, Morris has discussed about certain attitudes toward death and suicide

In India,[36] death is not final, but one incident in a long series of existences. It can, however, be regarded as timely or untimely, and suicide comes into the latter category. Untimely death is believed to be associated with an earth-bound ghostly after-life. He notes that death in India is regarded not as a solitary act, but as a part of the series of domestic rites and ceremonies in which not a single individual but whole families are required to play their several parts—"the Indian attempt to allay the anxieties universally occasioned by the threat of death." Recalling the thesis of Emile Durkheim on the causation of suicides and the inter-relation of social influences and individual abnormalities of behavior, Morris thought that the traditional caste-regulated Hindu society may protect individuals from suicide to some extent. However, he predicted that "It seems very likely that in India, in the next generation, we shall see an accelerated disorganization of the old-established sanctions, as the caste system is thrust aside in the process of economic Westernization. Already in the cities of India there are signs of that dilapidation of social values which Durkheim called anomie and according to his hypothesis one must predict a great increase in suicide, emotional instability, and crime. It will be interesting to see whether this will be borne out, or whether the Indian genius will succeed in adapting itself to the change with less disastrous consequences than the West has shown."

Development of Psychiatry in Low-income Countries

With his familiarity of India, having carried out his social anthropology field work in Rajasthan, Morris had a first-hand knowledge of the problems of mental health care in developing countries such as India. He delivered the Morison Lecture at the Royal College of Physicians of Edinburgh in May 1972 on "psychiatric problems of developing countries"[13] where he drew attention to the large contribution of mental disorders to chronic disability even in developing countries. In developing countries, because of the huge scarcity of psychiatrists, he called for the participation of general practitioners and government-employed general medical officers in providing mental health care, following short refresher course in mental health care. Subsequently, Morris assisted the WHO in promoting the training of basic health workers in rural areas of developing countries to identify, support, and provide care for seriously mentally ill and persons with epilepsy at primary healthcare centers.[37] It was realized that provision of mental health care through trained doctors and basic health workers in rural areas required large scale investments of training, organization, and supervision.

From 1968 to 1972, as the President of the World Federation for Mental Health (WFMH), an international, multi-professional nongovernmental organization (NGO), including citizen volunteers and former patients, founded in 1948 in the same era as the United Nations (UN) and the WHO, Morris contributed to the development of psychiatric facilities in developing countries, all over the world.[38] Morris was concerned about the place of psychiatry in medical education in developing countries and worked toward improving the status of psychiatry teaching for medical students.[39] Toward the end of his academic life in 1978, Morris contributed a couple of years to development of clinical services and training in psychiatry in three leading medical institutions in India.[40]

CURRENT STATUS

Psychiatric care and training have changed considerably since the period of 1950–1980, the three decades when Morris was academically active. Mental health care has moved beyond the deinstitutionalization movement to balanced care between general hospital psychiatry units, community, and nonhospital residential facilities. A new era of trans- and/or reinstitutionalization has begun. From a limited range of medications for psychiatric disorders during Morris's time, we now have a plethora of various types of psychopharmacological agents. Parallel revolutions in basic neurosciences and genetics of mental disorders have contributed to an abundance of new knowledge and understanding about various aspects of psychiatric disorders. However, most of the issues and problems that Morris had initiated research on continuing to be very relevant even today.

Some of Morris's initial interests and research were the need and significance of regular and useful work/employment for rehabilitation of the seriously mentally ill, the need for continued social supports for the discharged patients and their family members, and the influence of family on the course of severe mental illness. Morris also believed in the importance of social factors in the causation and management of mental disorders. Although the major focus of research in psychiatry during the past few decades was on biological aspects and the search for newer and more effective drugs, many leading biological psychiatrists have in recent years begun to recognize the importance of social factors. For example, Sir Robin Murray, writing about the mistakes that he had made in his research career noted: "I ignored social factors for 20 years. My preconceptions had made me blind to the influence of the social environment".[41] Tom Insel, former director of the National Institute of Mental Health (NIMH), USA from 2002 to 2015 who spent all his research years in biological psychiatry, said in his recent book, "Healing" that "Nothing my colleagues and I were doing addressed the ever-increasing urgency or magnitude of the suffering millions of Americans were living through... and dying from". He discovered that the cures for the crisis of care in America are not just medical but social and relational approaches.[42] Critically reviewing the narrowest of biological approaches that academic psychiatry is pursuing, Kleinman[43] argues for urgent rebalancing of academic psychiatry. He says: "what is required is rebalancing of the psychiatric academy to include greater support for researchers conducting social, clinical, and community studies."

The World Health Organization's current flagship program, mhGAP (Mental Health Gap Action Program) being implemented in many low- and middle-income countries across the world is aimed to scale up services for mental, neurological, and substance use disorders.[44] "Task shifting" is the process whereby specific mental healthcare-related tasks are moved, where appropriate, to health workers with shorter training and fewer qualifications in the community such as basic health workers.[45] Another similar term used is "task sharing" given to redistribution of care in the community to individuals with less or no formal training. These are continuations and expansion of Morris's prescription for development of mental health services in developing countries.

Morris was an ardent advocate for improving the quality and extent of psychiatry education for medical students and for appropriate postgraduate training for psychiatrists. Adequate and quality education and training in psychiatry both at undergraduate and postgraduate levels are important issues in most countries across the world. The content and duration of undergraduate and postgraduate training is highly variable across regions and countries contributing to wide variations in the nature and quality of mental health care.[46,47] With continuing crisis in recruitment to psychiatry in some countries and a global mental health workforce crisis, many of the recommendations made by Morris are still very valid.

CONCLUDING REMARKS

George Morrison Carstairs was a quintessential social, epidemiological, and community psychiatrist whose ideas and work were much ahead of his times. He was an empathetic clinician, an influential teacher, an able administrator, a prolific writer, an eloquent orator, an effective researcher and above all, an inspiring leader, and a role model. Morris was a lively and warm man of great social congeniality. Batches of psychiatrists and psychiatry trainees not only at the University of Edinburgh but also from many other countries, importantly from developing countries (including the author) immensely benefitted by their association with him in various capacities, from his kindness and generosity. As he was born and raised (his initial years) in India by his Scottish missionary parents, Morris had a special love for India and Indians. Indian psychiatry and psychiatrists have over the years reaped the fruits of this special relationship.

REFERENCES

1. Goffman E. Asylums: Essays on the Social Situation of Mental Patients and Other Inmates. New York, Doubleday: Anchor Books; 1961.
2. Barton WR. Institutional Neurosis. Bristol: Wright; 1959.
3. Brown GW, Wing JK. A comprehensive clinical and social survey of three mental hospitals. Sociol Rev. 1957;5:145-72.

4. Gruenberg EM. The social breakdown syndrome—some origins. Am J Psychiatry. 1967;123(12):1481-9.
5. Faris RE, Dunham HW. Mental Disorders in Urban Areas. Chicago: University of Chicago Press; 1939.
6. Srole L, Langner TS, Michael ST, Opler MK, Rennie TAC. Mental Health in the Metropolis: The Midtown Manhattan Study. New York: McGraw-Hill; 1962.
7. Leighton DC, Harding JS, Macklin DB, MacMillan AM, Leighton AH. The Character of Danger: Psychiatric Symptoms in Selected Communities. New York: Basic Books; 1963.
8. Carstairs GM. Obituary. Br J Sp Med. 1991;25(3):116.
9. News & Views. Psychological Medicine in Edinburgh: Professor GM Carstairs. Nature. 1960;188:984.
10. Rollin HR (Ed). George Morrison Carstairs. Psychiatric Bulletin. 1991;15:519-20.
11. Carstairs S. Vera Carstairs Obituary. The Guardian 4th January, 2021.
12. Carstairs GM. Research in social psychiatry. Scott Med J. 1961;6:391-6.
13. Carstairs GM. Psychiatric problems of developing countries. Based on the Morison lecture delivered at the Royal College of Physicians of Edinburgh, on 25 May 1972. Br J Psychiatry. 1973;123(574):271-7.
14. Carstairs GM, Tonge WL, O'Connor N, Barber LE. Changing population of mental hospitals. Br J Prev Soc Med. 1955;9(4):187-90.
15. Carstairs GM, O'Connor N, Rawns Ley K. Organization of a hospital workshop for chronic psychotic patients. Br J Prev Soc Med. 1956;10(3):136-40.
16. Carstairs GM. Some new initiatives in occupational therapy. Br J Occup Ther. 1958;21(6):14-6.
17. Carstairs GM, Heron A. The social environment of mental hospital patients: A measure of staff attitudes. In: Greenblatt M, Levinson DJ, Williams RH (Eds). The Patient and the Mental Hospital. Glencoe, Illinois: Free Press; 1957.
18. Brown GW, Carstairs GM, Topping G. Post-hospital adjustment of chronic mental patients. Lancet. 1958;2(7048):685-8.
19. Brown GW, Monck EM, Carstairs GM, Wing JK. Influence of Family Life on the Course of Schizophrenic Illness. Br J Prev Soc Med. 1962;16(2):55-68.
20. Wing JK, Monck E, Brown GW, Carstairs GM. Morbidity in the Community of Schizophrenic Patients Discharged from London Mental Hospitals in 1959. Br J Psychiatry. 1964;110:10-21.
21. Carstairs GM, Bruhn JG. Sociological Studies of Psychiatric Outpatient Practice. Sociol. Rev. 1957;5 (1_suppl), 91-115.
22. Royal Commission on Medical Education. Br Med J. 1968;2(5597):109-11.
23. Carstairs GM, Walton HJ, Smythies JR, Crisp AH. Psychiatric education. Survey of undergraduate psychiatric teaching in the United Kingdom (1966-1967). Br J Psychiatry. 1968;114:1411-16.
24. WHO Expert Committee on Mental Health & World Health Organization. (1963). Training of psychiatrists: twelfth report of the Expert Committee on Mental Health [meeting held in Geneva from 25 September to 1 October 1962]. [online] Available from https://iris.who.int/handle/10665/37993 [Last accessed February, 2025].
25. Carstairs GM, Brown GW. A census of psychiatric cases in two contrasting communities. J Ment Sci. 1958;104:72-81.
26. Kessel N. Self-poisoning. I. Br Med J. 1965;2(5473):1265-70.

27. Kessel N. Self-poisoning. II. Br Med J. 1965;2(5474):1336-40.
28. Carstairs GM. Characteristics of the Suicide-Prone. Proc R Soc Med. 1961;54(4):262-4.
29. Carstairs GM. Some Targets for Future Epidemiological Research. In: Hill D, Carstairs GM, Cartwright A (Eds). Burden on the Community, the Epidemiology of Mental Illness: a Symposium. London: Oxford University Press; 1962.
30. Carstairs GM, Kapur RL. The Great Universe of Kota: Stress, Change and Mental Disorders in an Indian Village. Berkeley: California University Press; 1976.
31. Diagnosis of a Sick Society. Br Med J. 1963;1(5324):135-6.
32. Carstairs GM. This island now. Br Med J. 1963;1(5324):141-6.
33. Carstairs GM. The Twice-Born: A Community of High Caste Hindus. London: Hogarth Press; 1957.
34. Carstairs GM. Hinjra and Jiryan: Two derivatives of Hindu attitude to sexuality. Br J Med Psychol. 1956;29(2):128-38.
35. Carstairs M. Medicine and faith in rural Rajasthan. In: Benjamin P (Ed). Health, Culture, and Community: Case Studies of Public Reactions to Health Programs. New York: Russell Sage Foundation; 1955. pp. 104-34.
36. Carstairs GM. Attitudes to Death and Suicide in an Indian Cultural Setting. Int J Soc Psychiatry. 1955;1(3):33-41.
37. Baasher TA, Carstairs GM, Giel R, Hassler FR (Eds). Mental Health in Developing Countries. Geneva (Papers presented at a WHO Seminar on the Organization of Mental Health Services, Addis Ababa, 27 November to 4 December 1973). Geneva: World Health Organization; 1975.
38. Carstairs GM. World Federation for Mental Health: a new regime. Am J Psychiatry. 1968;124(11):1573-4.
39. Carstairs GM. Psychiatry in basic medical education. In: Baasher TA, Carstairs GM, Giel R, Hassler FR (Eds). Mental Health in Developing Countries. Geneva: World Health Organization, 1975.
40. Carstairs GM. Development of psychiatric care in India. Bull R Coll Psychiatry. 1980:146-8.
41. Murray RM. Mistakes I have made in my research career. Schizophr Bull. 2017;43(2):253-6.
42. Insel T. Healing: Our Path from Mental Illness to Mental Health. New York: Penguin Press; 2022.
43. Kleinman A. Rebalancing academic psychiatry: why it needs to happen - and soon. Br J Psychiatry. 2012;201(6):421-2.
44. World Health Organization (WHO). mhGAP Intervention Guide. 2.0. Geneva: World Health Organization; 2019.
45. World Health Organization (WHO). Task shifting: rational redistribution of tasks among health workforce teams, Global Recommendations and Guidelines. Geneva: World Health Organization; 2008.
46. Isaac M, Ahmed HU, Chaturvedi SK, Hopwood MJ, Javeed A, Kanba S, et al. Postgraduate training in psychiatry in Asia. Curr Opin Psychiatry. 2018;31(5):396-402.
47. Gupta S, Menon V. Psychiatry training for medical students: A global perspective and implications for India's competency-based medical education curriculum. Indian J Psychiatry. 2022;64(3):240-51.

CHAPTER 10

Norman Sartorius

Debasish Basu

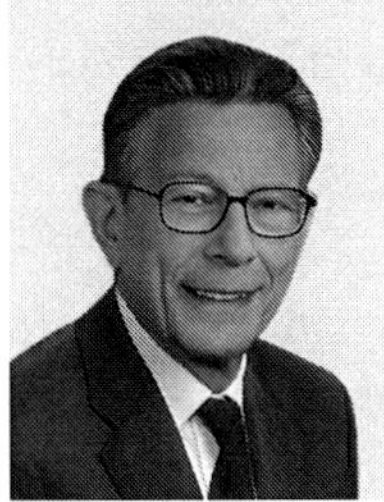

(Born - 1935)

INTRODUCTION

The latter half of the 20th century, especially the 1960s onward, was an interesting turning point for psychiatry, perhaps better called "crossroads." This era witnessed several challenges as well as opportunities. Psychiatry, while still largely institutionalized, with its coercive and rights-denying practices, also started witnessing the gradual spread of psychological and psychoanalytic-oriented therapies, some initial flickers of community-based practice, and the initial powerful wave of then new-generation psychopharmacology. However, psychiatric diagnostic and treatment practices still varied very widely across settings, countries, and continents. Mental illnesses were still heavily stigmatized, and so were the psychiatrists, often marginalized both within and outside the medical profession. It needed a great deal of work to make psychiatry—and psychiatrists and related mental health professionals—useful, scientific, compassionate, and respectable.

Against this backdrop, Norman Sartorius (1935 to present) emerged as a figure who took up the challenges. Over a period of six decades, especially the defining era of the 1970s and 1980s, through a brilliant series of multinational multicultural epidemiological studies conducted by the World Health Organization (WHO), he and his team contributed to the meeting of these challenges and turning them into opportunities.

Professor N Sartorius, MD, PhD, FRCPsych, previously the Director of the Mental Health Program of the WHO and President of the World Psychiatric Association (WPA) and of the European Psychiatric Association (EPA), now

TABLE 1: Notable publications.*

- Fighting for Mental Health (2002)
- Psychiatry in Society (with Gaebel W, Lopez-Ibor JJ, Maj M, 2002)
- Understanding the Stigma of Mental Illness: Theory and Interventions (with Arboleda-Flórez J, 2008)
- Ethics in Psychiatry (with Helmchen H, 2010)
- Paradigms Lost: Fighting Stigma and the Lessons Learned (with Stuart H and Arboleda-Flórez J, 2012)
- Comorbidity of Mental and Physical Disorders (with Holt RIG and Maj M, 2015)
- Paradigms lost, Paradigms Found – Lessons learned in the Fight Against the Stigma of Mental Illness (with Stuart H, 2022)

*These are a few important books written or edited by Sartorius, which are more relevant to this title. The total number of his scholarly publications is more than 500, and more than 120 books or book chapters.

serves as President of the Association for the Improvement of Mental Health Programmes (AIMHP), a nongovernmental organization located in Geneva, Switzerland. Professor Sartorius holds several professorial positions in Europe, the USA, and elsewhere. He has published more than 500 papers in peer-reviewed journals and authored, coauthored, edited or coedited more than 120 books. More details on his publications follow later.

Professor Sartorius' main areas of interest at present are the comorbidity of mental and physical disorders, the reduction of the stigma of mental disorders and education of psychiatrists and other stakeholders in the field of mental health. In his previous positions, he was the principal investigator of a number of international collaborative studies and projects dealing with schizophrenia and other major mental diseases, comorbidity of mental and physical illnesses, health service development, and education of different categories of staff.

The lifelong work of Professor Sartorius spans more than six decades (his first scientific publication was in 1961,[1] and still continuing with the latest publication in June 2024[2] at the time of writing this chapter in the same month); it has covered virtually all aspects of psychiatry—biological, pharmacological, clinical, nosological, epidemiological, technical, social, ethical, public health, advocacy, leadership, training, and preventive. From this ocean, a few major trends are reflected in this chapter which are in keeping with the scope and mandate of this book. A few notable books written or edited by him are shown in **Table 1**.[3-9]

BRIEF BIOGRAPHY

Norman Sartorius was born in Germany in January 1935 where his mother, Dr Fedja Fischer Sartorius, a well-known pediatrician and enthusiast in mother and child health promotion, worked at the time.[10-16] She was also an Associate Professor, Director of Croatian Center for Maternal and Child Health, Zagreb, Croatia. His father, F Sartorius, was a medical doctor and Professor of Public Health at the University of Münster, Germany. However, due to the increasingly discriminatory effects of Nazism in German society, Norman's mother found it progressively difficult to continue her professional work in Germany. Further, his parents underwent divorce, following which he returned with mother to Croatia in 1938. Thus, at Norman's age of 2-plus, he with his mother came to Croatia (her parents' home country), which was then a part of the Kingdom of Yugoslavia, and he started elementary school in a provincial town there. Then World War II broke out, when Norman was barely 7–8 years old. His mother joined the Yugoslavian resistance against the German occupiers and their local helpers, and they spent "the subsequent war years in the forests and provinces of Croatia where we experienced war at its worst."[4] They survived the ordeal, and at the end of the war, came to Zagreb, the capital, where he completed secondary school in 1952. He then went to the medical school in Zagreb, largely because of family expectations that the elder of the children should take up medicine so that there is a doctor in the next generation.

Norman became Doctor Sartorius in 1958 in Zagreb, one of the youngest medical graduates at 23 years of age. He did not want to go to pediatrics because his mother was already a famous figure in pediatrics, and he did not take up his then favorite ophthalmology because that was too coveted a subject usurped by those with political clout. He instead went for an unpaid volunteer placement in psychiatry, initially. He shuddered at his experience in the psychiatric ward the very first day of his joining when he saw patients waking up after induced insulin coma, screaming. However, he stuck to the training, and, after completing training for the title of a specialist of psychiatry and neurology (which were still the same specialty at the time in 1963), he continued studies to obtain an MA and PhD in psychology from the faculty of Psychology in 1964. He was interested in psychology because it provided information about normal psychological functioning and about research methods both of which were not covered very well by the graduate training in psychiatry.

In 1965, Dr Sartorius obtained a British Council scholarship and spent the next 20 months in England where "I made friendships that last to this day and learned a lot, particularly about doing research in psychiatry." In all ways, these 20 months proved transformative in his career. He fondly recalls his appointment with Sir Aubrey Lewis (which he sought as he was initially unhappy with what he was doing there—he was told it would be a very short interview, but it lasted 2 hours and was a fascinating experience for the young trainee), which opened the doors for exposure to a broad and exciting vista of psychiatric knowledge and research.

In 1967, Dr Sartorius joined the WHO to work on epidemiological and social psychiatry, starting from the famous International Pilot Study of Schizophrenia (IPSS). Thus started his association with the WHO, an association that would last for 27 years. In 1973, he became the Head of the Mental Health Unit of the WHO; the Unit was elevated to the level of an Office of Mental Health in 1975 and in 1977 it finally became the Division of Mental Health, of which he was the first Director until 1993. After this, he left the WHO to take a professorial post at the University Department of Psychiatry in Geneva, and later at other universities. Much of the work that he did at the WHO was done in the field, and during his years at WHO, he usually spent a third of the year traveling to the many countries that participated in WHO's mental health program or expressed their intention to do so.

Professor Sartorius also had professorial appointments in several other universities in the USA (St Louis, New York, University of Florida), the UK (London), China (Beijing), Czech Republic (Prague), France (Paris), Croatia (Zagreb and Osijek), and Serbia (Belgrade) and he was honored by doctorates, awards, and fellowships in other countries. In 1993, he was also elected President of the WPA (1993–1999), and in the year 2000, President of the EPA. Soon after that, in 2004, he and colleagues created a nongovernmental, not-for-profit organization the AIMHP (https://aim-mental-health.org/), of which he continues to be the President. AIMHP's objective is to make a contribution to the improvement and promotion of mental health programs worldwide. It aims to achieve its goals by means of consultation, by organizing talks and seminars, by initiating and coordinating studies, and other theoretical and practical work, and by any other appropriate means that can improve the care of people with mental illness and their families and raise the value given to mental health by individuals and societies.

During his professional career Professor Sartorius published more than 500 papers in peer reviewed journals and more than 800 technical contributions—prefaces to books, interviews, and brief articles. He has also authored, coauthored, or edited more than 120 books. According to Google Scholar, as of this writing (June 2024) Professor Sartorius' articles have been cited more than 80,000 times; his h-index is 118, i10-index is 492; he has 16 articles with more than 1,000 citations each. According to ResearchGate, he has 938 publications, nearly 400,000 reads (on ResearchGate itself) and nearly 50,000 citations.

In recent years, Professor Sartorius has focused his attention on the reduction of stigma of mental illness, on comorbidity of mental and physical disorders and on support to carers of people with mental disorders. He has been particularly interested in the education of young professionals and conducted leadership and professional skills courses in some 60 countries involving more than 3,000 psychiatrists early in their career.

Regarding his personal life, he has two half-brothers. His wife, Vera, MA engineering, MA Egyptology and Classical Archeology, is a historian. They have one daughter, Danielle, who is a medical doctor (anesthesiologist) living in Geneva with her medical internist husband. He also has two lovely grandchildren, girls aged 11 and 16 years.

MAJOR CONTRIBUTIONS

It is very difficult, if not impossible, to list and provide details of the professional contributions of a person of the stature of Norman Sartorius, whose active psychiatric career has spanned more than six decades, within the space restraints of this chapter. An attempt is made here to summarize his widely varying contributions to psychiatry in the following areas: (1) Assessments and epidemiology; (2) nosology; (3) cross-cultural psychiatry; (4) services, especially integration of mental health care with primary health care; (5) comorbidity of mental and physical illnesses; (6) training and leadership in psychiatry; and (7) stigma. Many of his initial contributions to psychiatry happened during his 27-year stint with the WHO, continuing with his later years with WPA, EPA, and now AIMHP.

Assessments and Epidemiology

In more than one sense, the contributions of Norman Sartorius are to be seen as inseparable from the contribution of WHO in the area of mental health from the mid-1960s till the early 1990s, not surprisingly because of his pivotal role in the WHO.

The WHO program on epidemiology of mental disorders started in the early 1960s with a series of reviews of knowledge. These were followed by activities aiming at four main goals: The standardization of psychiatric diagnosis, classification, and statistics; the development of standardized internationally applicable instruments for the assessment of mental patients and of variables relevant to the assessment of mental illness; the conduct of epidemiological studies of mental disorders; and the training relevant to the above goals.[17]

The first and undoubtedly one of the most important contributions of Sartorius, with lasting value even after nearly six decades, was his role as the principal investigator of the nine-country IPSS.[17,18] This was a pioneer psychiatric epidemiological study in all senses, covering a broad sweep of developed and "developing" (now called low- and middle-income) countries: Colombia, Czechoslovakia, Denmark, India, Nigeria, China, (then) Union of Soviet Socialist Republics, the United Kingdom and the United States of America. The initial evaluation phase of the IPSS demonstrated that it is possible, using standardized reliable methods of assessment, to identify schizophrenic patients in centers in nine countries of the world, who are similar with regard to their clinical picture at the time of a psychotic episode. Furthermore, it demonstrated that the symptomatology of these patients was different from the symptomatology of patients with other functional psychoses. These findings have important implications for many types of research into schizophrenia, since they indicate that genetic, epidemiological, psychopharmacological, and other studies of schizophrenia can be carried out in a fashion that will ensure reproducibility of results. The demonstration that it is possible to identify symptomatically similar schizophrenic patients across diverse cultures in a reliable fashion was an important step forward in attempts to understand more about the nature of schizophrenia.

There have been many previous follow-up studies of schizophrenia. The follow-up phase of the IPSS was unique, however, in allowing a description of the course and outcome of a large number of people with schizophrenia who were prospectively selected in several different parts of the world and reassessed and evaluated in standardized fashion. Sartorius and others concluded that, in summary, the IPSS developed standardized, reliable, and internationally applicable instruments for psychiatric assessment; it demonstrated the feasibility of large-scale international transcultural psychiatric studies; it provided material and operational methodology for carrying out such studies; it provided methods of analyzing large amounts of data and procedures for training investigators in the use of standard techniques; and it enhanced basic knowledge about the nature of schizophrenia and other functional psychoses. The large patient sample that has been assessed in a standardized fashion in nine countries served as a reference group for future studies.[17,18]

Very importantly, the IPSS has also resulted in the creation of a network of research centers in economically and socioculturally contrasting countries. In these centers, there are now research workers trained and experienced in transcultural psychiatry who have established working relationships with one another and who have indicated a desire to continue their study of transcultural and psychiatric problems. This network-building capacity led to a large number of multinational, multicentric studies on various aspects of epidemiology: Schizophrenia, depression, acute psychoses, dementia, psychological problems seen in general healthcare, and other mental and neurological illnesses with mental health implications.

It also helped to develop a number of important assessment instruments which could be used across countries and cultures: Instruments for assessing diagnosis, disability, quality of life, and many others. Assessment methods that have been produced through the program are of demonstrated applicability and reliability in different cultural settings. They span the entire field of psychiatric disorders and psychosocial problems. Centers that have participated in the production of these instruments and methods have, in many instances, become repositories of information and training sites for new users. These have been invaluable in conducting future studies.

Nosology

Right from the early years, when there was the International Classification of Diseases (ICD) 7th edition, there was a felt need to improve the nosology and diagnostic practices, which were shown to be grossly inadequate in the famous US-UK diagnostic project. Sartorius contributed importantly in the production of 8th revision of the ICD (ICD-8), ICD-9, and later ICD-10. A step forward in the development of the classification was that his team succeeded to introduce glossary definitions in the text of the ICD-8 which improved its use. The ninth and then the 10th revision had also been accompanied by separate volumes containing definitions of each category of the classification.

In preparation for the 10th Revision of the ICD (ICD-10), a major program was launched in the early 1980s. The classification of mental disorders in ICD-10 is presented in several versions. The version for clinicians was translated into 13 languages. Several other versions were prepared, including the diagnostic criteria for research accompanying the ICD-10 classification of mental disorders, a version for primary care, a version for child mental disorder, and a multiaxial presentation of the classification. In each instance, the release of the version was preceded by a field test of the proposals. Many centers participated in the testing of the version for the clinicians' centers. A large number of people with mental disorders were examined and jointly rated by psychiatrists in the tests of the clinical and research version of ICD. Similar exercise was undertaken for tests of the other versions. The classification was tested and released in several languages and a network of centers has been established to help or train users and monitor the experience obtained in the use of the classification.

After this major contribution, he has later been involved with providing consultation for the development of ICD-11 and the American Psychiatric Association's Diagnostic and Statistical Manual 5th edition as well.

Cross-cultural Psychiatry

Right from the beginning of Sartorius' involvement with WHO, the efforts were on recruiting centers from diverse settings (urban and rural) in diverse countries (developed and low- and middle-income) among diverse cultures and populations. By the time he left WHO, it was involved with mental health related work with more than 60 countries. IPSS showed the seeds of important cross-cultural work in nine countries. This was followed by many other works between 1967 till 1993:[17] Some examples being later studies on schizophrenia (24 countries), depression (11 countries), acute psychoses (12 countries), dementia (eight countries), psychological problems in general health care (12 countries), neurological disorders (eight countries), disability (seven countries), and mental disorders in HIV-affected individuals (six countries). Cross-cultural involvement has been instrumental also in the development and standardization of the many assessment instruments and in the classificatory studies especially for ICD-10.

Overall, "in looking back at WHO's program in epidemiological psychiatry over the past 25 years, three achievements seem to be particularly worthwhile: First, the contribution that the program has made to knowledge on mental health and mental illness in different sociocultural settings; second, the contribution that the program has made to the development of methods that allow the conduct of national and cross-cultural comparative and collaborative studies; and third, the fact that the program has created a worldwide network of individuals and centers willing and able to work together. It is this last success that is closest to WHO's true role of an agency whose role is to help people of the world to work together in improving health and human understanding worldwide."[17]

Services

Another major contribution of Sartorius and his teams spread all over the world is the area of service development and evaluation. From his early days as a student in psychiatry in Zagreb through his early days as a researcher posted by the WHO in India, Sartorius was struck by the lack of adequate services for the mentally ill in many ways and the necessary need to improve upon the services in innovative ways, given the seemingly unsurmountable gap between demands and resources available. Under his stewardship, WHO embarked on a number of multicountry studies to plan and improvise services catering to various aspects of mental healthcare needs. These included community response to alcohol problems, psychological support for those undergoing sterilization, public health problems linked to use of psychotropic drugs, the "pathways to care" studies, and multiaxial recording of problems in general health care.

However, of all these studies, the study aiming at the assessment of *strategies for the extension of mental health care*[19] was undoubtedly the most influential in terms of changes in mental health programs in WHO member states. The study had several phases. During the first phase, an epidemiological study of mental disorders was undertaken to obtain baseline data and to use them in designing training programs. After that, health workers in each of the study areas participating in a study received brief task-oriented instruction on the detection and management of mental disorders that were particularly frequently seen in the area. Training about a number of interventions involving community agents, such as teachers, police, communal leaders, village chiefs and in some cases, traditional healers, was then undertaken. The areas were evaluated again after the training of health workers had been completed to establish the impact of such training. This study was later extended to six further centers; as in the first batch of countries, it produced interesting data and had a significant impact on health decision makers in the areas, which allowed the use of the results of the study in designing community-based mental health services. This study paved the path for formulation of mental health policies and programs in many countries, by demonstrating that mental healthcare can be successfully integrated with general health care at the primary health care settings.

Comorbidity of Mental and Physical Illnesses

Another persistent area of Sartorius's contribution has been his emphasis to bring psychiatry closer to mainstream medicine, in order to reduce its marginalization and alienation, which in turn is one of the important ways to reduce stigma against psychiatry and psychiatrists (see later). As a part of this endeavor, it is important to study, document, and treat comorbidity between mental and physical illnesses. Further, the life expectancy of people with mental illness grew but they are still dying 10–15 years sooner than the rest of the population. Providing care for physical illness in people with mental illness has therefore emerged as a main problem for health services in the 21st century. Sartorius has been involved with several multicentric multinational studies in this area, especially those of diabetes. He and his coauthors started by a production of a series of books that brought together existing evidence and should serve as the basis for action programs. The books published so far cover physical illness and schizophrenia; intellectual disability and health; physical illness and drugs of abuse; depression and diabetes; depression and heart disease; and depression and cancer, among others. His involvement in this area is evident from the fact that he initiated and helped to develop the INTERPRET-DD, which is a 14-country study on epidemiology of diabetes and depression, One of the recent publications with data from 12 countries concluded: "The importance of psychosocial factors in addition to physiological variables in the development of depressive symptoms and incident major depressive disorder (MDD) in people with type 2 diabetes. Stressful life events, depressive symptoms, and diabetes-related distress all play a significant role which has implications for practice. A more holistic approach to care, which recognizes the interplay of these psychosocial factors, may help to mitigate their impact on diabetes self-management as well as MDD, thus early screening and treatment for symptoms is recommended."[20] The study produced a number of papers showing that people who suffer from diabetes frequently have depressive disorders which are not recognized nor offered treatment.

Training and Leadership in Psychiatry

Another major contribution of Sartorius is his long-lasting passion in providing professional training and leadership skills to especially early career psychiatrists. It is not surprising that through his very long and active professional life he has had ample opportunities to train many generations of students. What sets him apart is his continued commitment to this area. As he writes, one of his areas of ongoing interest is "to manage and lead the series of courses on leadership and professional skills for young psychiatrists in various countries. These are very intensive and require a lot of preparation but are continuing to delight me because they are offering me a chance to meet many young people with vast talent and creative power in many countries and to remain optimistic about the future of psychiatry."[8] Such programs have been conducted in around 60 countries over a period spanning more than three decades. People who attended these programs describe them as enriching and unforgettable experience.

Stigma

This section has been kept at the end of the "major contributions", not because of any hierarchical considerations. Indeed, this remains another active pursuit area of his interest and has been so for the past many decades. This is one area which pertains directly to social psychiatry, and in which Sartorius has been vocal in many forums as evidenced by his publications over three decades. He has authored several important books on stigma related to psychiatric disorders, some of which are mentioned in the "notable publications" **(Table 1)**. Indeed, as WPA President in 1996, he embarked on an ambitious project called "Open the Doors." It was an international initiative to fight the stigma and discrimination associated with schizophrenia. Since then, the "Open the Doors" program has been implemented in more than 20 countries and has involved more than 200 interventions aimed at reducing stigma against individuals with schizophrenia.

As Sartorius said in his Yves Pelicier lecture at the World Congress of Social Psychiatry, Bucharest, October 2019, "There are good news and bad news about stigma related to mental illness. The bad news is that stigma is still attached to mental illness and to all that touches it–mental health services, psychiatrists and mental health workers, psychotropic medications, families of those suffering from mental illness and other people providing care, institutions in which people with mental illness are treated, and any treatment offered to people who have a mental illness. The good news is that recent years have seen the development of national and regional programs aiming to reduce stigma in many countries—in Australia, Brazil, Canada, the Czech Republic, Denmark, England, Hong Kong, Germany, Ireland, Japan, the Netherlands, New Zealand, Portugal, Scotland, Singapore, and Wales."[21]

However, despite excellent programs against stigma that have started in some countries, he recognized that in most countries of the world stigma of mental illness is still not effectively tackled. The main reason for this is that the paradigms which have been the basis for national efforts to combat stigma are no longer valid so that progress now depends on developing and applying approaches different from those used so far. With his huge experience and wisdom, Sartorius recommends "that the programs against stigma should be directed at well-defined groups of people and that it should be preceded by an exploration of their views and situations in which they will meet people with mental illness. Work against stigma should not be conducted by "campaigns" but become a routine part of the program of health services, planned, permanent, and funded like any other vital function of the service. In antistigma programs, efforts to increase mental health literacy should follow the acquisition of practical skills enabling people to understand and work with people suffering from mental illness. Social contact with people who experienced mental illness is a powerful tool for the reduction of stigma. The goal of antistigma programs should be a change of *behavior* concerning mentally ill people, not only a declaration of changed attitudes. The evaluation of the success of antistigma programs should be searched in improvements of laws concerning mental illness, in rates of employment of people with mental illness, in their acceptance in the community, in housing, and opportunities for participation in community life. The ultimate goal of antistigma programs should not be that communities tolerate those who are mentally ill but that they include them and treat them as they would any other member of the community."[21]

CURRENT STATUS

Given this broad overview of the wide-ranging work of Professor Norman Sartorius, one might wonder, why is his name being included in this "Twelve beacons of light in *social* psychiatry"? In other words, what is his status in—and his contributions toward—social psychiatry?

The answer might initially be baffling, because Sartorius himself is not a great fan of "social psychiatry" as a sub/superspecialty area of psychiatry. Indeed, some years ago, he made a tongue-in-cheek comment: He wrote that social psychiatry will "disappear" and that it is likely that "the world will be a slightly better place without it"! However, as he clarified the issue in the preface of a book named "Psychiatry in Society" which he edited:

> *The reason for this statement was that it is unimaginable that psychiatry could be practiced or that psychiatric research could be conducted without constant reference to social factors and to the social environment. It was agreed that it is therefore unnecessary to have social psychiatry as a special discipline—all psychiatry being also social—but it is also harmful to use this term because the existence of social psychiatry could be taken as a proof that good psychiatry can exist without its social component.*

Sartorius immediately further emphasized: "The changes of the social context affect the incidence and prevalence of mental disorders, their course and outcome, and their reaction to treatment. Social changes are also of determinant importance for the rehabilitation of people who had mental illness. They affect, furthermore, the organization of health care, the training of healthcare staff, and the willingness and capacity of families to look after their sick members."[4]

Elsewhere, he gives another amusing yet instructive anecdote regarding the use (or, rather, avoidance) of the term social psychiatry in the 1960s–1970s: "Emphasizing social factors and social psychiatry was dangerous for one's career in some countries where "social", "socialist" and related words were an indication of communist leanings: Senator McCarthy's court cases in the USA and other symptoms of the cold war touched psychiatry as well. Thus, for example, the first meeting of the World Association for Social Psychiatry in London in 1964, was convened at the same time and in the same city as another "biologically oriented" meeting: Colleagues from the West who attended the social psychiatry meeting were not telling others that they attended it. Similarly, but for different reasons, Eastern European psychiatrists were avoiding social psychiatry possibly to remain respected by the majority of psychiatrists in their countries with prevailing biological orientation in psychiatry."[11]

Norman Sartorius, though averse to calling himself a "social psychiatrist", and generally disapproving of creating artificial dichotomies and divisions within psychiatry, has consistently highlighted the "social" in all aspects of psychiatry, not as a psychiatric sub/superspecialty but as a quintessential element. His lifelong crusade against stigma of mental illnesses can be seen as a major contribution to social psychiatry. Other "social" components inherent in his thoughts, activities, and publications can be exemplified in a few brief exemplars below.

A New Definition of Mental Health

In an expanded and revised concept of mental health, it was defined by the authors (which included Sartorius) as: "Mental health is a dynamic state of internal equilibrium which enables individuals to use their abilities in harmony with universal values of society. Basic cognitive and social skills; ability to recognize, express and modulate one's own emotions, as well as empathize with others; flexibility and ability to cope with adverse life events and function in social roles; and harmonious relationship between body and mind represent important components of mental health which contribute, to varying degrees, to the state of internal equilibrium."[22] They further elaborate "universal values of society" as "respect and care for oneself and other living beings; recognition of connectedness between people; respect for the environment; respect for one's own and others' freedom."[22] As is evident, this entire definition places the human being, and their mind, in the context of the society and defines mental health from this vantage point.

Culture/Society in Relation with Psychiatric Diagnosis, Clinical Features, Treatment Seeking, and Outcome

The entire life's work of Sartorius—starting from his contribution to the US-UK diagnostic project, IPSS and all the later studies on schizophrenia, depression, acute psychoses, pathways to care studies, and others bear testimony to this assertion. Examples, galore, have been chronicled earlier.

Community Care

Rampant urbanization, commodification of mental healthcare service, excessive and at times mindless digitalization of society, and a thinning concept of "community"—all these have impacted the traditional community care. Sartorius has recently proposed a set of important changes in care in the community to be effective in this new era. This is "principles of social psychiatry" directly in action. However, he also cautions that "The suggestions made here may require a significant reorganization of services, and an investment into the training of personnel who will provide care, of persons experiencing mental illness, and of their carers. It is also clear that it is necessary to provide services with financial resources which are at present lacking in most parts of the world. This may be seen as or declared as impossible at present—if such is the case, it will be necessary to realize that it is extremely unlikely that fiddling with arrangements without the provision of additional resources will producc solution to the current crisis of community care for people with mental illness, their families, and other carers."[23]

Caring for the Carer

The abovementioned trends in the society not only impact the patient but their carers as well. The wearing out of the traditional social network (the real, in-person network—not the virtual "social media" network though it might be better than having none at all) particularly adversely affects both instrumental/logistic support as well as emotional/cognitive support of the carers. Sartorius in his recent talks has been focusing on this area as a focal point that needs urgent attention. Indeed, this has been identified as an area of new priority for mental health programs of the future in his recent "Lifetime Recognition Oration" delivered at the Diamond Jubilee International Conference of Mental Health held in Chandigarh, 14–16 September 2023.[24]

Preventive Psychiatry, Promotion of Mental Health

Public health principles have been core to many of the WHO activities. However, traditionally the focus has been on treatment of already established mental illnesses rather than thinking in terms of preventing these. The epidemiological studies of the WHO did combine clinical psychiatry with public health principles. A number of activities and programs can be undertaken as preventive-promotive activities, again underlined as a key priority area for new mental health programs. Many of these would require a population based, public health approach, and many would overlap with social psychiatric principles—public mental health, social determinants of mental health, social epidemiology, stigma of mental illness and how to address it, community care, and fostering healthy communities.[24]

Ethics, Rights, Social Justice

Finally, ethics, human rights, and social justice for the persons with lived experience of mental health conditions is slowly gaining traction as a long-neglected area. Sartorius has written about it in his recent publications. "The concepts of human rights, social justice, and social determinants of health are inextricably intertwined with public health. Globally, attention is increasingly being paid to the connections between social determinants and the challenges of sustainability, well-being, and justice. Social factors and socioeconomic inequities are among the root causes of many public health problems. Yet, research in psychiatry over the past few decades has paid insufficient attention to their impact and focused its main attention on neuroscience research and biological models. Health authorities emphasized the need to develop algorithmic approaches for patient care, paying little attention to the social contexts of health care. In this article, we highlight the complementary relationship between human rights, social justice, social determinants, and public mental health. We argue that the promotion of the mental health of the population requires protection and promotion of economic and social rights and equitable access to resources and opportunities."[25] In this context, it is pertinent to mention that the updated second edition of "Ethics in Psychiatry" (a book edited by Sartorius and his colleagues) is about to be published soon.[26]

CONCLUDING REMARKS

Professor Norman Sartorius has enriched psychiatry in all aspects, including its social aspects, with his tireless work over six decades. Very rightly he has been called "Psychiatry's living legend".[15] Much earlier, in 2003, while reflecting on his book "Fighting for mental health: A personal view," Professor Simon Wessely considered him as one of the most famous psychiatrists of all time.[16] Accolades are not new for Professor Sartorius, with dozens of honorary or distinguished Fellowships from professional societies, honorary or visiting professorships at universities, honorary degrees or decorations from associations, including at least three lifetime achievement awards. However, perhaps more than anything else, he is regarded for his Course on Leadership and Professional Skills for Early Career Psychiatrists, mentioned above. A Letter to the Lancet Psychiatry, published by 47 of his students apropos to the Living Legend article, characterized Sartorius as: "To conclude, Sartorius's wisdom, openness, kindness, high standards of knowledge, truly humanistic values, creativity, honesty, and great sense of humor are just a few of his attributes that have made him an outstanding mentor, inspiring teacher, and motivating leader. If only workforce development and education were always done in the same manner, accessible and available to more people in ours and others' professions, we would live in a different world where mental health is not only a discipline, but a part of everyday life for all. Sartorius is indeed a living legend with a legendary heritage of people, who have been trained by him, who are devoted to his work, and believe in the future where nobody is left behind, be it patients or professionals."[14]

REFERENCES

1. Sartorius N. Prva klinicka iskustva sa preparatom Trilafon (Clinical experience with Trilafon). Neuropsihijatrija. 1961;9:335-40.
2. Okasha T, Mostafa BM, Ibrahim I, Abdelgawad AA, Lloyd CE, Sartorius N, Elkholy H. Comorbidity of depression and type 2 diabetes in Egypt results from the International Prevalence and Treatment of Diabetes and Depression (INTERPRET-DD) study. Int J Soc Psychiatry. 2024;70(4):730-8.
3. Sartorius N. Fighting for Mental Health. Cambridge: Cambridge University Press; 2002.
4. Sartorius N, Gaebel W, Lopez-Ibor JJ, Maj M. Psychiatry in Society. Chichester: John Wiley & Sons; 2002.
5. Arboleda-Flórez J, Sartorius N (Eds). Understanding the Stigma of Mental Illness: Theory and Interventions. Chichester: John Wiley & Sons; 2008.
6. Helmchen H, Sartorius N (Eds). Ethics in Psychiatry. International Library of Ethics, Law, and the New Medicine. London: Springer; 2010.
7. Stuart H, Arboleda-Florez J, Sartorius N. Paradigms Lost: Fighting Stigma and the Lessons Learned. London: Oxford Academic; 2012.
8. Sartorius N, Holt RIG, Maj M (Eds). Comorbidity of Mental and Physical Disorders. Basel: Karger; 2015.
9. Stuart H, Sartorius N. Paradigms lost, Paradigms Found – Lessons learned in the Fight Against the Stigma of Mental Illness. Second Edition. Oxford: Oxford University Press; 2022.
10. Norman Sartorius. In: Bhugra D (Ed). Psychiatrists on Psychiatry: Conversations with Leaders. Chapter 19. Oxford: Oxford University Press; 2023. pp. 180-90.
11. Norman Sartorius Interview. (2021). RAD 548. Medical Sciences 56-57 (2021):174-85. [on line] Available from https://hrcak.srce.hr/file/392279 [Last accessed February, 2025].

12. Sartorius N. Notes of a traveller. Acta Psychiatr Scand. 2011;123(4):239-46.
13. Sartorius N. Norman Sartorius: a personal history of psychiatry. Global Psychiatry. 2020;3(1):1-8.
14. Krupchanka D, Pinto da Costa M, Jovanović N; 47 individuals. Norman Sartorius: psychiatry's living legend. Lancet Psychiatry. 2019;6(12):983-4.
15. Lane R. Norman Sartorius: psychiatry's living legend. Lancet Psychiatry. 2019;6(10):811-2.
16. Wessely S. Norman Sartorius: a champion of mental health. Lancet. 2003;361:709.
17. Sartorius N. WHO's work on the epidemiology of mental disorders. Soc Psychiatry Psychiatr Epidemiol. 1993;28:147-55.
18. Sartorius N, Shapiro R, Jablensky A. The International Pilot Study of Schizophrenia. Schiz Bull. 1974:1(11):21-34.
19. Sartorius N, Harding TW. The WHO collaborative study on strategies for extending mental health care, I: the genesis of the study. Am J Psychiatry. 1983;140(11):1470-3.
20. Lloyd CE, Sartorius N, Ahmed HU, Alvarez A, Bahendeka S, Bobrov AE, et al. Factors associated with the onset of major depressive disorder in adults with type 2 diabetes living in 12 different countries: results from the INTERPRET-DD prospective study. Epidemiol Psychiatr Sci. 2020;29:e134.
21. Sartorius N. Fighting Stigma 2020: Synopsis of the Presentation of the Yves Pelicier Prize Lecture at the World Congress of Social Psychiatry, Bucharest, October 2019. World Soc Psychiatry. 2020;2:181-3.
22. Galderisi S, Heinz A, Kastrup M, Beezhold J, Sartorius N. Toward a new definition of mental health. World Psychiatry. 2015;14(2):231-3.
23. Sartorius N. Community care for people with mental illness: challenges emerging in the 2020s and consequent recommendations. World Psychiatry. 2023;22(3):388-9.
24. Sartorius, N. (2023, September). *The mental health workforce of the future: Qualities and tasks*. Lifetime Recognition Oration presented at the Diamond Jubilee International Conference of Mental Health, Chandigarh, India.
25. Sartorius N, Gill N, Virani S, Salvador-Carulla L. Fighting for human rights and social justice and the promotion of mental health: Complementary efforts. World Soc Psychiatry. 2023;5:97-100.
26. Helmchen H, Gather J, Sartorius N (Eds). Ethics in Psychiatry. Berlin: Springer; 2024.

Ravi L Kapur

Roy A Kallivayalil, Rakesh K Chadda

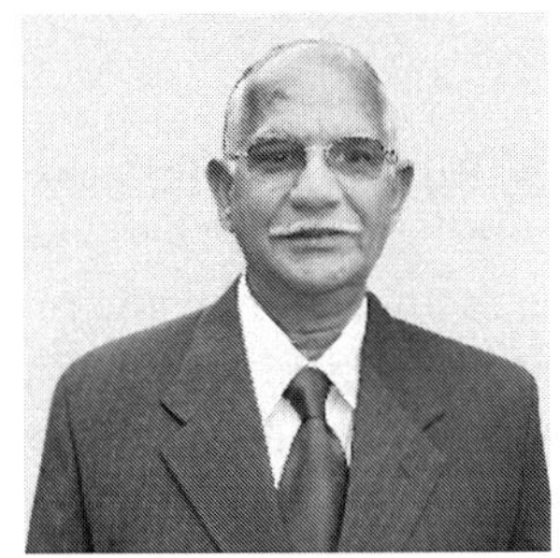

(1938–2006)

INTRODUCTION

Ravinder Lal Kapur was a colossus in Indian psychiatry, an original thinker, and a professor extraordinary. He came from a rare breed of psychiatrists who were trained in India when postgraduate training in psychiatry had just begun. He went to the United Kingdom a short while after qualifying in psychiatry from India and returned to India after a few years and contributed to the growth of psychiatry in a unique manner. In his initial years after returning from the United Kingdom, Kapur worked in psychiatric settings in a medical school and a neuroscience hospital. Afterward, he was involved in social science research, diversifying from the main field of psychiatry. Kapur had made immense contributions to Indian psychiatry, including psychiatric epidemiology, social and community psychiatry, school mental health, postgraduate training in psychiatry, qualitative research, and diverse social issues, including violence and terrorism **(Table 1)**.

BRIEF BIOGRAPHY

Kapur was born on July 7, 1938, in Lahore, currently in Pakistan. His father, Dr Mohan Lal Kapur, was a general practitioner and was highly regarded in the professional and social circles in Lahore. The family had to migrate from Lahore to Delhi in the summer of 1947 during the historic partition of India by the British into independent India and Pakistan. His parents were able to escape from Lahore, taking him along on one of the last trains leaving Lahore

TABLE 1: Notable publications.

- The Great Universe of Kota (1976)
- Kapur, R. L. (1995). *The Great Universe of Kota: Stress, Change and Mental Disorder in an Indian Village*. Sage Publications.
- Indian Psychiatric Interview Schedule (1974)
- Indian Psychiatric Survey Schedule (1974)
- The role of traditional healers in mental health care in rural India (1979)
- Community involvement in mental healthcare (1994)
- Violence in India: A psychological perspective (1994)
- Qualitative methods in mental health research (1999)
- Another Way to Live (2009)

for Delhi just before the new Pakistani border was closed. His four sisters had been able to migrate to Delhi earlier. At Delhi, his elder sisters were often taking care of him. During the partition, while migrating to Delhi, all their family's belongings had been left behind in Lahore. The 9-year-old Kapur was also a witness to the explosive violence on the streets. These events had an important impact on the molding of his personality. He was to study the genesis of violence in the country in the later years of his life.[1]

Kapur joined medicine at the Government Medical College, Amritsar, and finished his graduation in 1960. Though he joined the MBBS course, he was reluctant to be a doctor, as his general practitioner father had wished him to be. He was very good in studies but wanted to be in theater as an actor. His father expected him to excel in his studies and not to waste time on trivial activities. During his medical studies, he often showed interest in the artistic life in Delhi. He also had a keen inclination toward cinema, art exhibits, and meeting creative people. However, his father's pressure made him continue in medicine.

Dr JS Neki, a well-known psychiatrist and renowned poet (who later became Director, Postgraduate Institute of Medical Education and Research, Chandigarh), taught him psychiatry during MBBS. Dr Neki persuaded him to take up psychiatry so that he could combine his interest in theater and in the healing profession.

Just after finishing his MBBS, Kapur worked as an assistant surgeon at the Government Mental Hospital, Amritsar, from January to June 1961. Here, he worked under the legendary Dr Vidya Sagar, famous for treating patients with families in tents outside the premises of the main hospital building. In 1963, he joined the All India Institute of Mental Health (AIIMH) [now National Institute of Mental Health and Neurosciences (NIMHANS)], Bangalore, and finished his diploma in psychological medicine (DPM) in 1965 with a distinction. Subsequently, he worked as a lecturer in psychiatry for about a year (August 1965–August 1966) at the Medical College, Baroda.[2]

After working in psychiatry at three different settings (north, south, and west) in India, there was a major turning point in his career when he got selected for the Commonwealth fellowship. He worked as a Commonwealth medical fellow under GM Carstairs in the Department of Psychiatry, University of Edinburgh, from October 1966 to October 1967, and subsequently continued as a research assistant at the same place. The work at Edinburgh also earned him PhD from the university. While at the University of Edinburgh, he was also designated as honorary lecturer in psychiatry from December 1966 to January 1972. After coming back to India, he was instrumental in setting up the Department of Psychiatry at the Kasturba Medical College, Manipal (1974–1975). In October 1975, he was appointed as Professor of Community Psychiatry at NIMHANS, Bangalore, where he worked till October 1983, and also headed the department of psychiatry from June 1976 to April 1983.[2]

After leaving NIMHANS, Kapur joined the Indian Institute of Science (IISc), Bangalore, where he worked from April 1983 to August 1985 as a consultant psychiatrist and visiting professor at the Center for Theoretical Studies in the Center for the Study of the World Religions. In September 1985, he moved to Harvard University as a Fulbright scholar in residence and visiting professor in the Department of Social Medicine and the Center for the Study of World Religions. He finished his tenure at Harvard University in June 1986. Thereafter, he joined as a consultant in mental health for Somalia at the World Health Organization (WHO) Eastern Mediterranean Region, Alexandria, where he worked for about 4 months from July to October 1986. Later, he served as professor of psychiatry at the National Institute of Advanced Studies (NIAS) at the IISc, Bangalore, from October 1988 to January 1998, and continued as Emeritus Professor till his death. For about 6 years, from February 1990 to March 1996, he also served as Deputy Director, NIAS, IISc Bangalore campus.

In the period of 1985–2000, Kapur conducted many psychosocial studies on a wide range of topics, including creativity among Indian scientists, the psychological profile of terrorists in Punjab and Kashmir, the psychological roots of violence, and the alienation of youth in the country. During this period, he had also conducted a study on the psychological and social characteristics of the *sanyasis* (holy men) living in the Himalayas. The study was supported by the Indian Council of Medical Research (ICMR) and included visiting the *sanyasis* in remote locations in the Himalayas, including Rishikesh, Gangotri, and Badrinath. Kapur's work was recognized by many scientific societies, and he was elected fellow of many prestigious scientific and professional bodies, including the National Academy of Medical Sciences of India, the Royal College of Psychiatrists of the United Kingdom, and the Indian Academy of Sciences, Bangalore.

Kapur got married to Malavika Karanth (Kapur) on April 24, 1965. Malavika Kapur is now an honorary professor at the NIAS, Bangalore. Earlier, she had served as Professor and Head, Department of Clinical Psychology at the NIMHANS, Bangalore. She has several books and over 100 papers to her credit. They have two children, daughter Svapna Sabnis, a pediatrician, and son Sharad Kapur, a mathematician. They also have four grandchildren.[3]

Just before his death, Kapur had gone as "scholar in residence" of the Rockefeller Foundation at the Villa Serbelloni on Lake Como, Bellagio, Italy, to write his book "Another Way to Live" based on Indian sadhus. Unfortunately, he passed away of cardiac arrest there on November 24, 2006. He had presented his work to the other scholars on the previous day. His wife Malavika writes, "He had wanted me to promise to fulfill two of his wishes. One is that he should die a quick and painless death and secondly that he should die before me!" His wife was on his side when he died. Prior to his demise, he had mailed all his family and friends that he was most happy in the extraordinary, beautiful surroundings of Lake Como with extensive gardens. It was as if his life's mission had been accomplished in writing "Another Way to Live."[3]

Kapur had many accolades and honors that he hardly noticed, but his pride was in the creation of the NIAS, Bangalore. His greatest disappointment was in not getting appointed as the Director of the Institute as Dr Raja Ramanna (founder Director) intended him to be. But it was not to be so. JRD Tata and Raja Ramanna treated him like their own son and had great fondness for him.[3]

Kapur was an intense and risk-taking person. Empathy was his strong and weak points. He would become overinvolved with his patients, but he believed that one could truly reach another person only through deep empathy. He was widely read in a great number of fields, be it philosophy, literature, performing arts, or scientific endeavors. On the surface, it appeared that he took life easy, light hearted, and fun loving. Surprisingly, his family members, his sisters, and nephews, with whom he had intense emotional bonding, had no clue about his versatility with the wide range and depth of his interests as well as achievements. He loved his children and grandchildren to distraction.

MAJOR CONTRIBUTIONS

Kapur's areas of interest varied from psychiatric epidemiology, social and community psychiatry, and school mental health to qualitative research connecting spirituality, psychology, and psychotherapy. In later years of his life, he had become interested in research on diverse social issues, including violence and terrorism, an area that had bothered him since his childhood days, when he was witness to the massive violence of 1947, the partition of British India into India and Pakistan.

Psychiatric Epidemiology

Kapur's interest in epidemiology started from his stay in Edinburgh, where he got familiar with the basic principles of the field. In February 1970, he, along with his wife Malvika Kapur, began the Edinburgh–Manipal Psychiatric Research Project, conceived in 1968–69 during his stay at Edinburgh under the stewardship of Professor GM Carstairs. He was the field director of the project. The site of the study was a small village, Kota, a coastal community located north of Mangalore and 18 miles from Manipal in the state of Karnataka in South India. The project had been started on the lines of the Stirling County study and the Midtown Manhattan study, which were conducted in Canada and the United States of America, respectively, in the 1960s. One of the biggest challenges for the study was developing a study instrument, which would be feasible to use in the local population. The challenge involved measuring and comparing the impact of change and stress on mental disorders among the three main cultural groups (Brahmins, Bants, and Mogers) living in the Kota community.[4]

The study had two bases of operations in India, AIIMH (now NIMHANS), Bangalore, and the Kasturba Medical College, Manipal, for conducting the research. Two instruments, the Indian Psychiatric Interview Schedule (IPIS) and the Indian Psychiatric Survey Schedule (IPSS), were developed for conducting the study.[5,6] IPSS included 125 psychiatric symptoms and included commonly found symptoms in the Indian population. The phrasing of the questions was done in simple language which could be easily understood by the villagers. IPIS and IPSS were used to assess the prevalence of psychiatric symptomatology among the local population. Both the questionnaires were translated into Kannada under the supervision of Malavika Kapur, a clinical psychologist by profession and well versed with the local language. IPSS was applied to 50% of the population in all three groups.

Investigators had also recorded the religious beliefs and practices of three communities, as well as the functioning of the caste systems and the family patterns. The study found a kind of historical change in the family pattern with the family hierarchy gradually shifting from a traditional matrilineal system to a patrilineal structure. There were also differences observed in religious practices between the three communities. While the Brahmins would worship the major gods of the Hindu religion, most of the Kota villagers were primarily worshippers of lesser spirits or bhutas (ghosts), who were also identified by their names and authorities in the local area. Agriculture, fishing, and local commerce were the common sources of income. A large number of subjects admitted having psychological symptoms as assessed on IPIS and IPPS. Thirty-two percent of men and 40% of women reported one or more symptoms. Most of the villagers having emotional distress would be managed by a caring approach from the families and local healers. The study took nearly 3 years to collect the data. The final analysis and report writing were done at Edinburgh. The report was finally published in the form of a book, The Great Universe of Kota: Stress, Change, and Mental Disorder in an Indian Village.[4]

Community Psychiatry

The Edinburgh–Manipal Psychiatric Research Project was an important initiative, which brought focus on community mental health in India. Kapur, after joining the NIMHANS, took community mental health as one of his priority areas of work. Holding a professorial position in community psychiatry, the first in the country, he did full justice to this role. In his critical approach to the community mental health movement, which was promoted in India, he always kept in mind what he learned during the Kota study of the early 1970s as guiding principles. He disagreed openly with mental health planners who were turning a blind eye to the abundant traditional healing resources available in communities, particularly in rural areas.[7,8]

When, on August 6, 2001, 28 chained inmates of a home for mentally ill died, as they were unable to escape the fire that engulfed the thatched shed in Erwadi of Ramanathapuram district, Tamil Nadu, Kapur went against the liberal and progressive minds who were asking to close down such religious facilities. He reminded the health administrators that these institutions were actually providing daily support to many chronic patients and their families and that such sheltering institutions should be offered financial support and supervision rather than closure. He had learnt from the Kota study that villagers remained loyal to their traditional representations of mental disorders and to their healers, though they were open to new knowledge and remedies that could prove to be helpful.

In an important critique in 1994, Kapur[7] narrated the story of the community mental health movement in India, criticizing most of the plans put into action in the country, particularly the National Mental Health Programmes (NMHP). NMHP was started in 1982 with the ambitious aim of ensuring availability and accessibility of minimum mental health care for all. Kapur's critiques hit the NMHP at the very heart: The objectives set were "extremely unrealistic"; the approach was "top-down" and did not take into account the ground realities. Further, a lack of enthusiasm and "poor morale" had weakened the functioning of the primary healthcare approach; the absence of a solid administrative structure led to the failure of the NMHP in most health districts of the country.

Kapur was convinced that there were various ways to provide cheap, manageable, and efficient services for mentally ill patients in India. For common mental disorders, the role of folk healing, spiritual and religious counseling, and ancient techniques (like yoga) was to be promoted. Quite provocatively, he wrote, "Is going to spiritual healers worse than doling out expensive tranquilizers under the pressure of various drug companies?"[8] For more severe mental troubles, he repeatedly proposed that specialized professional services should be offered, such as training for general practitioners, nurses, psychologists, and social workers. These specialists could then better synchronize their activities with those of psychiatrists, either in hospitals or in the community. This proposal could not work out in more explicit terms and never served as a model for building a community-oriented psychiatry in India.

Kapur tirelessly promoted a socially and culturally grounded psychiatry over four decades.[9] In a critical commentary on the Diagnostic and Statistical Manual of Mental Disorders III (DSM-III), he argued eloquently against the conceptual uniformity that such a diagnostic manual imposes on all mental health practitioners, wherever they work around the world. He proposed that psychiatrists should rather look for the processes which are behind symptoms and signs, for it is in learning about these processes that the meaning of distress experienced by the patient needs to be assessed.[10]

Clinical Psychiatry

For 8 years (1974–1982), Kapur was Professor of Community Psychiatry and Head of the Department of Psychiatry at the NIMHANS, Bangalore. He never wanted to create his own school or to have disciples or hangers-on groupies. Many of his former students remember him as one of the most creative thinkers, contributing to the consolidation of linkages between social sciences, psychology, and psychiatry in the development of an Indian psychiatry. He will certainly be remembered in the history of Indian psychiatry as a key figure who consistently promoted a culturally and phenomenologically oriented psychiatry. This was in opposition to the dominant biological and neurological approaches, which have invaded Indian psychiatric research and practice. Kapur walked a solitary path in his constant exploration of himself. He was often dissatisfied with his own achievements, requesting always more and more of himself and striking a fine balance between intellectual independence and social engagement. Students and young researchers who worked with him remember him as a demanding master who always pushed them ahead with a firm hand. His commitment to the development of an Indian style in psychiatry transformed him into an inspirational thinker who sometimes took the attire of a visionary rebel.

Although he interrogated continuously the role of spirituality in the practice of psychotherapy, he remained a personification of secularism to which he brought a new meaning: He could sing classical Hindustani ragas or Indian classical music of north India, listen to the poetic Ghazals, and read the Bhagavad Gita, the Koran, and the Bible with equal interest. He found in all these texts some answers to the questions he posed about the way to be human.[3]

In his essay on "What is psychotherapy?" he outlined the meaning of therapy for him: Life is nothing but a bundle of contradictions, and a therapist must realize that there are never going to be final answers to some questions. For example, how much should the therapist involve himself with the patient? If you do not involve yourself, you are often not effective; if you overinvolve yourself, you get transference problems. A therapist must walk on the razor's edge between these polarities. The psychotherapy Ravi practiced was quite paradoxically informed by the Indian spirituality that tells the patient to "dis-identify with the ego" and the Western-style psychology that rather aims "at the strengthening of the ego." Here again, Kapur, the therapist, walked on the razor's edge in combining what certain orthodox minds may judge contradictory. For him, the essence of psychotherapy was "an affectionate and respectful relationship" and not the "excavation" of the so-called truth hidden behind the patients' problems. At a more substantive level, he tried to anchor his clinical practice in the Hindu ideas of selfhood and personhood, ideas that should stand, according to him, at the very center of any Indian style of psychotherapy.

During his stay at NIMHANS, he developed a team of young researchers, with work on diverse areas like psychiatric morbidity among graduate and research students,[11] postpsychotic depression,[12] cost-effectiveness analysis of different methods of psychiatric care,[13] community models of care,[14] a comparative clinical trial of electroconvulsive therapy (ECT) and imipramine in depression,[15] psychiatric morbidity in general practice,[16] and reactive psychosis.[17] Thus, he inculcated research aptitude in many young psychiatry trainees, who went on to be leaders in the field.

Above all, Kapur was a clinician who was fully dedicated to his patients: They could call him anywhere and anytime, and he was always ready to chat with them, whatever he was doing at the moment of the call.

Understanding Yoga

From 1981 to 1982, he took sabbatical leave (awarded by the ICMR) to spend a year as an apprentice disciple (*sadhaka*) with a guru, a yoga expert. He had decided to move away from his usual research on epidemiological studies of large populations to concentrate on "the study of only one person," namely himself. During his year-long retreat, he underwent intensive training in yoga and studied, at the phenomenological level, the impact of mental exercises, meditative disciplines, and other yoga techniques on his personal mental state. In a personalized experience, he wanted to confirm whether or not yoga techniques actually induced psychological well-being in individual practitioners. In addition, he wanted to ascertain if these practices brought about feelings of joy, energy, harmony, alertness of mind, detachment, and eventually an enriched inner life. Thus, he himself was the subject of this self-experiment in which he submitted himself to a long-term personal experience of yoga practices under the close supervision of a guru. He systematically recorded, on a daily basis, any change in his own mental state, emotions, and inner life. After completion of this experience, he tried to identify the consistent patterns, which were present in the daily notes and observations of his diary. He was highly influenced by Patanjali (the ancient Indian yoga guru). Two main reasons may explain this. First, he recognized himself in the deep atheism of this thinker whose philosophy establishes linkages between nature (prakriti) and self (purusha), the cosmic and psychological realities, and the body and the mind. In Patanjali's philosophy, the realization of one's own infinite *Atman* in its identification with *Brahma* is achieved without any reference to religion: The God *Shiva*, the Supreme Yogi, is never present at the horizon. The second reason was that he shared with Patanjali several ideas regarding the way to achieve liberation (*moksha*) from instinctual drives, compulsive desires, and fluctuations of mind.

Sociopolitical Issues

Kapur engaged in a joint project with colleagues of the Schizophrenia Research Foundation (SCARF) at Chennai. With them, he wanted to explore the contribution of culture to the trajectory of people with psychosis. The group was particularly interested in investigating the ways religion and spirituality could allow a particular elaboration and culturalization of the posture of "positive withdrawal," which has been suggested to be protective for people with psychosis in North America.[18,19] Kapur proposed that "positive withdrawal" could be a proxy for the well-spread notions, across India, of distance, detachment, and renunciation that are key elements in the Indian definition of selfhood. The study focused on asceticism, considered as a readily available cultural idiom on offer to people confronted by a range of limit experiences, possibly including psychosis. In collecting life trajectories of *Sadhus* and *Sanyasis*, Indian ascetic figures, it was proposed to map the degree of flexibility of the language of renunciation, its appropriation or distortion by individuals, and its transformative power. The researchers met different kinds of persons who were confronted with the limits of experience. In parallel with the study, which was continued with the SCARF collaborators, Kapur continued research with persons engaged in an ascetic quest for spirituality (*Sadhus and Sanyasis*) and people coming to consult them. They conducted interviews with walking *Sadhus and Sanyasis*, including the ones living in ashrams. The intention was to pay particular attention to individuals situated "at the borders" of the life of renunciation: At its internal borders, for people living an extreme form of detachment that could be read as a mark of their special status on the pathway to knowledge; at its external border, for extremely marginal and solitary people who could be eventually encountered in pilgrimage centers, in *Anna Kshetras* (feeding places for walking Sadhus and poor people), or on the roads. It was assumed that among individuals bearing the marks of *Sadhuism,* some might be eventually trapped in a psychotic-like state, the language offered by *Sadhuism* being either a way to contain their problems or a sort of escape that made possible a culturally acceptable marginal lifestyle.

With Kapur's departure, we realize how privileged we have been to have him as a guide in the clarification of some of our intuitions and ideas in research and in our explorations of the spiritual dimension of India. We will keep forever the memory of all these years of working together, chatting and arguing, debating on sensitive issues, and enjoying walking in the Himalayan foothills. We owe to Kapur an immense enrichment of our vision of life: He introduced us to the inner face of Indian society and culture; he allowed us to meet exceptional people; he always reminded us of the necessity to combine rigor, empathy, and creativity. And indeed, we shared with him so many ideas, hypotheses, and visions; the passion to discover, to learn, and to discuss the refusal to idealize whatsoever, understanding spirituality as a trademark of India, and the rejection of all sorts of exoticization. Passionate discussions with him constantly nourished our interactions and our work, adding to the precious character of our relationship.

Kapur had a deep commitment for whatever he did, his intelligent grasp of complex matters, and his passionate quest for truth that led him sometimes to explosive positions during debates. He always showed deep humanity in his interactions. The following vignette borrowed from one of his accounts illustrates well his great humanity: "*Three Sadhus came together into the Ashram at the afternoon tea time. They politely asked the kitchen staff whether they could sit down and have tea. I was watching them and liked their comradeship, their laughing and joking. It is never easy to start off a conversation with strangers but I felt it would be interesting to talk to them. So, I went over, told them I was a psychologist and was interested in knowing what led them to Sanyasa and in what way they had changed after taking Sanyasa. After one of them had disappeared, I invited the two others into my room, gave them two chairs to sit on and myself sat on the ground.*"[20] Just imagine the scene: Kapur is seated cross-legged on the floor while the two *Sadhus* sit on the chair. Questions could then begin: "So how did you go into *Sanyas*?" asked Kapur. The above vignette shows the atmosphere of trust and respect that Kapur was able to create and thus the quality of the interviews with Sadhus he did and later discussed.

Violence in Society

Questions related to violence accompanied Kapur all whole life: "Why did Hindus, Muslims and Sikhs who had lived peacefully together for decades begin to kill one another?"; "How were communities so rapidly transformed into battlefields of conflicting loyalties?"; "Why were the long traditions of tolerance and non-violence so ineffective in containing the explosions of religious fanaticism?"; "What sort of poison dissolved the morality of communities and contaminated individuals to the point of transforming them into killers of their neighbors, friends and even family?" These questions permeated Kapur's intellectual life, which was dedicated, at least on one front, to understanding the human implications of the catastrophic historical event of 1947 that he had witnessed. During adolescence, he had recurrent nightmares during which he saw people being slaughtered in front of him. He was calmed by the presence of his loving elder sisters. He tried to escape this emotional pain through two strategies. First, by silence and cleavage: He refused forever to talk openly about what had happened during the train trip to Delhi; he avoided films or books dealing with the issue of partition; and he never took the opportunity to visit Lahore. He was hoping to do so for a 2007 meeting of psychiatrists between the two Punjabs, but anticipating this meeting stirred old memories. Almost 40 years after Partition, he was revisited by the nightmares of his adolescence, similar to this one he described in an article: "*I am walking on the road with friends. Four people catch hold of others walking on the road and mercilessly chop them with cutlasses. The bits and pieces of bodies are strewn all over. The others on the road just look and go away. I try to scream but my friends stop me, saying it will not help to scream. When I point out that what was happening was terrible and the killers must be punished, I am told that it would not help me to agitate because no one will respond. There is also a threat in the air that if I say anything I shall be the next victim. The assassins smile after the act—even laugh loudly and I cry with impotent rage.*"[21]

Qualitative Research

As the head of the Science and Society Unit at the NIAS, Kapur promoted research dealing with the creative process in science. In this study, he compared the mental processes of scientists and artists as they made discoveries or artistic composition with the mystical experiences of *Sanyasis*. Such a comparative frame resulted in a very original approach for the study of creativity among scientists. During his stay at NIAS, he also tirelessly promoted the place of qualitative research methods in all fields. This led him to conduct an important workshop with papers, which were published as a book in 1995.

CURRENT STATUS

Kapur made many important contributions to Indian psychiatry. His was one of the initial works in psychiatric epidemiology in the country which probably ran parallel to the International Pilot Study of Schizophrenia, in which India had a center in Agra. "The Great Universe of Kota" stands as an important testimony to the voluminous work carried out by him with GM Carstairs. The study, along with its two instruments, IPIS and IPSS, was a unique contribution at a time when conducting epidemiological research was a big challenge. This also serves as an important motivation for the young researchers.

Kapur had been a very popular teacher and stimulated his students in clinical research. Research conducted by his students under his guidance covered important contemporary areas like reactive psychosis, postpsychotic depression, ECT, and family burden. He also attempted developing linkages with the general practitioners with an important work on psychiatric morbidity in general practice, something unusual in the 1970s. As a professor of community psychiatry, he did full justice to his job by developing the community mental health unit at NIMHANS, Bangalore. His initiatives in community psychiatry were the forerunner of the NMHP of India, which was launched in 1982. In the 1990s, when the NMHP had not made much progress even after a decade of its launch, he wrote a very appropriate critical analysis outlining reasons for it not getting implemented in principle.

Kapur had also advocated involving the traditional healers in mental health care, since a large section of the population in India consults them for mental health issues. Thus, integrating them into mental health care might help in reducing the treatment gap. Many psychiatrists in later years have supported this approach.

His later work on qualitative research in mental health while at NIAS has stimulated many young psychiatrists to take up qualitative research. He also stands apart from many contemporary psychiatrists by taking up issues of sociopolitical violence, basically looking at its genesis and how such problems might be reduced. His experiments with spirituality were also attempts at understanding its role in mental health in the contemporary world.

To commemorate him, the RL Kapur Memorial Oration is being held every year at the NIAS, Bangalore. He had built the institution in its formative years as Deputy Director along with Raja Ramanna, who was the Director. The first RL Kapur memorial oration was delivered by Sudhir Kakar on August 23, 2013. Eminent scientists and thinkers have delivered this oration in subsequent years: Girishwar Mishra in 2014, Ashish Nandy in 2015, Manoj Das in 2016, Gilles Bibeau in 2017, Vijay Padaki in 2018, Chiranjiv Singh in 2019, BN Goswamy in 2022, Om Prakash in 2023, and Ravi Narayan in 2024. Though Kapur passed away in 2006, his legacy continues in the form of many important contributions in the field of mental health.

CONCLUDING REMARKS

Kapur was perpetually in search of truth and the meaning of life that eluded him. He was an atheist and a most rational person. He was a very complex person and had a layered persona, and he was a blend of rationality on one hand and empathy on the other. He was a risk taker even in terms of holding on to jobs. His travels in the Himalayas along with his wife Malavika and meeting the sadhus was one path he had traveled together with his wife for >25 years that resulted in the book "Another Way to Live." He will always be remembered for his unique contributions to social and community psychiatry in his first 20 years of professional life, when he decided to leave the core discipline of psychiatry to pursue his interest in understanding social issues like violence in society. Kapur will be remembered as a profound thinker and seminal figure in the fields of social and community psychiatry.

REFERENCES

1. Bibleau G, Corin E. Dr Ravi L Kapur (1938–2006): A psychiatrist at the crossroads of multiple worlds. Transcult Psychiatry. 2010;47:159-80.
2. Bhide A. Remembering a Giant. Indian J Psychol Med. 2006;28:6-7.
3. Kapur M. Personal communication on RL Kapur. 2024.
4. Carstairs GM, Kapur RL. The Great Universe of Kota: Stress, change and mental disorder in an Indian village. London: Hogarth Press; 1976.
5. Kapur RL, Kapur M, Carstairs GM. Indian Psychiatric Interview Schedule (IPIS). Soc Psychiatry. 1974a;9:61-9.
6. Kapur RL, Kapur M, Carstairs GM. Indian Psychiatric Survey Schedule (IPSS), Soc Psychiatry. 1974b;9:71-6.
7. Kapur RL. Community involvement in mental healthcare. Natl Med J India. 1994;7:(6):292-4.
8. Kapur RL. The role of traditional healers in mental health care in rural India. Soc Sci Med Med Anthropol. 1979;13B(1):27-31.
9. Kapur RL. Mental health care in rural India: a study of existing patterns and their implications for future policy. Br J Psychiatry. 1975;127:286-93.
10. Kapur R. Commentary on "Culture-Bound Syndromes and International Disease Classification." Cult Med Psychiatry. 1987;11:43-8.
11. Chandrashekar CR, Shamasundar C, Kapur RL, Kaliaperumae V. Mental morbidity among graduate and research students: an epidemiological study. Indian J Psychiatry. 1980;22:89-93.
12. Das P, Kapur RL. Post-psychotic depression in schizophrenics: (a prospective study). Indian J Psychiatry. 1980;22:277-82.
13. Isaac MK, Kapur RL. A cost-effectiveness analysis of three different methods of psychiatric case finding in the general population. Br J Psychiatry. 1980;137:540-6.
14. Isaac MK, Kapur RL, Chandrashekhar CR, Kapur M, Parthasarathy R. Mental health delivery in rural primary healthcare—Development and evaluation of a pilot training programme. Indian J Psychiatry. 1982;24:131-8.
15. Gangadhar BN, Kapur RL, Kalyanasundaram S. Comparison of electroconvulsive therapy with imipramine in endogenous depression: a double blind study. Br J Psychiatry. 1982;141:367-71.
16. Gautam S, Kapur RL, Shamasundar C. Psychiatric morbidity and referral in general practice-a survey of general practitioners in Bangalore city. Indian J Psychiatry. 1980;22:295-7.
17. Kapur RL, Pandurangi AK. A comparative study of reactive psychosis and acute psychosis without precipitating stress. Br J Psychiatry. 1979;135:544-50.

18. Corin E. Facts and meaning in psychiatry: an anthropological approach to the lifeworld of schizophrenics. Cult Med Psychiatry. 1990;14:153-88.
19. Corin E, Thara R, Padmavati R. Living through a staggering world: the play of signifiers in early psychosis in South India. In: Jenkins J, Barrett R (Eds). Schizophrenia, culture and subjectivity. Cambridge: Cambridge University Press; 2004. pp. 110-45.
20. Kapur R. Account of an encounter with a walking Swami. (unpublished manuscript). 2001.
21. Kapur R. Violence in India: a psychological perspective. Indian J Psychiatry. 1994;36:163-9.

Julian Leff

Tom KJ Craig

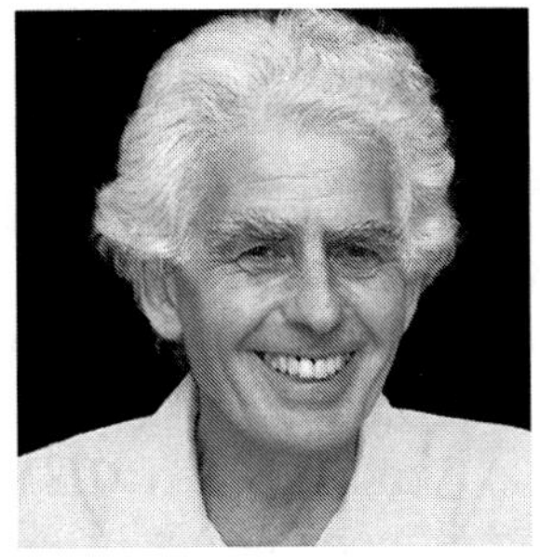

(1938–2021)

INTRODUCTION

In this tribute, I provide a brief synopsis of Julian Leff's surprisingly versatile research focusing mainly on schizophrenia. Much of his early work drew upon and extended the measures developed by colleagues at the Social Psychiatry Unit (SPU) at the Institute of Psychiatry in London. The unit aimed to investigate the social factors that led to persistent mental illness and disablement and to develop techniques of treatment and prevention. Among the important achievements of the unit were the development of the Present State Examination (PSE) a semi-structured interview used to measure psychiatric symptoms and the related CATEGO computerized classification program;[1] the Camberwell Family Interview (CFI)[2] and an early version of the Life Events and Difficulties schedule[3] used to assess the impact of stressful experiences in everyday life.

One of Julian's first tasks as a junior researcher was to assist in administering the PSE for the London center of the WHO international study of schizophrenia. Through this activity, he met many international colleagues and forged links that led to his involvement in the second WHO schizophrenia "Determinants of Outcome" study and to enduring links with the WHO. This international work fueled an interest in the cultural differences in how mental distress was experienced, whether it was seen to need special help (be that from traditional healers, "barefoot doctors" or medical practitioners) and what this help might involve, including the role of family and wider support networks. His books *"Psychiatry around the Globe"* and the *"The Unbalanced Mind"* (see notable publications in **Table 1**) deal in depth with these fundamental issues.

BRIEF BIOGRAPHY

Julian Paul Leff was born in London in 1938, the son of parents who had a profound commitment to social equity and to the welfare and health of the population. Both were members of the British Communist Party. They met in November 1936 tending to the blistered feet of men who had walked the 300 miles to Parliament from the Midlands. This famous "Jarrow March" was a defining moment in the social reform of British society. The march was an organized protest against the parlous conditions of poverty, unemployment, and rotten housing in the town of Jarrow in an industrial belt of North East England. It was one of a number of "hunger marches" organized by the National Unemployed Workers Movement, a communist led organization. Julian's father, Sam, a doctor and member of the Socialist Medical Association, helped to plan the National Health Service (NHS) that eventually came into existence in 1946. His commitment to social conditions and public health included serving as Medical Officer of Health for Willesden, and training as a Barrister to better argue the case for preventive medicine. Indeed, his conviction was so great he tried to dissuade Julian from becoming a doctor.

Julian's mother Vera, a poet and novelist, was similarly active in the social movement, involved with the campaign for Nuclear Disarmament. Sam and Vera wrote many books jointly on the importance of social conditions in the genesis and management health including, *From Witchcraft to World Health (1956), The School Health Service (1959), Health and Humanity (1960),* and *The Search for Sanity* which addressed issues of the social aspects of mental illness.

Julian qualified in medicine from University College London in 1961. He worked as a junior doctor at the Whittington Hospital and eventually came to psychiatry at the Maudsley Hospital in 1965. His intellect and talents obviously impressed his seniors so that he soon embarked on a career as a member of staff in SPU at the Institute of Psychiatry working alongside some of the founding fathers of modern psychiatry including John Wing, Jim Birley, Michael Rutter, and George Brown. Julian became the assistant director in 1974 and full director of the Unit when John Wing retired in 1989. He led a hugely productive and distinguished career producing >300 scholarly publications and 9 books. He received several notable awards including the Starkey Prize from the Royal Society of Health 1976; the Inaugural Burgholzl Award from the University of Zurich 1999; the Marsh Award for Mental Health Work 2010; Honorary Fellowship of the Royal College of Psychiatrists 2015; and the Yves Pelicier Lifetime Achievement Award from the World Association of Social

TABLE 1: Notable publications.

- Expressed Emotion in Families (Guildford New York, 1985)
- Psychiatry Around the Globe (Gaskell, London 1988)
- The Unbalanced Mind (Weidenfeld and Nicolson, London 2001)

Psychiatry 2017. Dubbed the "Attenborough of Psychiatry", Julian was a highly accomplished teacher, liked and respected by his many trainees in the UK as well as by those who came from overseas when he was Dean of foreign students at the Institute of Psychiatry. He lectured and taught on six continents, often accompanied by his wife, Joan Raphael-Leff (a distinguished psychoanalyst and transcultural psychologist), and children and led a happy and fulfilling family life. His many talents went far beyond psychiatry to include playing the piano, singing in a choir, silk printing, upholstery, ceramics, glassware, and the design and manufacture of silver jewelry.

Julian died peacefully at home after a long illness, on Tuesday February 23, 2021. He is survived by his wife, his four children (Alex, Jessa, Jonty, and Adriel), and nine grandchildren.

MAJOR RESEARCH CONTRIBUTIONS

It may come as a surprise, that one of first studies that Julian led was a controlled trial antipsychotic medication prevention of relapse in schizophrenia.[4] Aware of the work of Brown and Birley,[3] he included their measure of life events in this study and showed that most patients who relapsed despite medication had experienced one or more stressful life events in the 5 weeks before relapse[5] thus providing evidence of an interaction of biological and social factors.

In this rest of this chapter, I will focus on Julian's major research contributions, including family intervention (FI) in schizophrenia; the closure and reprovision of a hospital asylum; ethnicity, migration, and schizophrenia; and the invention of AVATAR therapy. All reflect his wider interest in the contribution of personal relationships in the onset and courser of schizophrenia.

Expressed Emotion and Family Intervention

The origins of Julian's pioneering work with the families of people suffering from schizophrenia go back to some of the early work of the Social Psychiatry Research Unit examining the outcomes of patients discharged from hospital. This showed a puzzling finding. Patients who returned to live with their parents had higher rates of relapse and readmission than those who lived with their siblings or were in private lodgings.[6] Thinking this might reflect difficulties in the emotional interaction between patients and their family carers, George Brown and Michael Rutter developed the CFI to assess the quality of the personal relationship between patient and family members[2] with measures of warmth, critical comments, hostility, and overinvolvement (the latter reflecting the extent of the relative's protectiveness, self-sacrifice, and mutual dependence). Relatives who scored highly on critical comments, hostility or overinvolvement were classified as showing high "expressed emotion (EE)". More than half of the patients who lived with a high-EE carer relapsed compared to just one in six of those in low-EE homes, while antipsychotic medication and reduced contact with high-EE relatives were protective.[7]

Julian took up these findings in further research, frequently conducted in the patients' own homes.

With his colleague, Christine Vaughn, he used a shortened version of the CFI and replicated the findings for high EE in relapse of schizophrenia. They showed the additive effect of medication use and time away from the high-EE family with patients on both regular medication and limited exposure to high EE having the lowest risk of relapse. Their study also included a group of patients who had recovered from severe depression. High EE was also relevant for this condition although the majority of patients lived with spouses so that overinvolvement was less frequent than in the work with schizophrenia, and the presence of just two critical comments discriminated between those who relapsed or did well implying even greater sensitivity to criticism.[8]

High EE echoed other investigations that showed people suffering from schizophrenia to be sensitive to the effects of stressful life events.[3] In a series of experiments with Nick Tarrier, arousal measured by skin conductance was captured for patients living in a high-EE home, patients in low-EE homes and a third group of healthy participants also living at home. While the conductance data was being recorded, participants spent 15 minutes sitting in a room with the researcher after which the relative was invited to join them for a further 15 minutes. Conductance was higher and similar for both EE groups compared to healthy participants during the first phase. In the second phase, when the patient's relative entered the room, those from high-EE homes had a much greater conductance response that was maintained without apparent habituation. In contrast, patients from low-EE homes showed rapid habituation like that seen in the healthy participants.[9]

It should be obvious that a social relationship concept such as high EE must, to some extent, be determined by cultural norms. While the original thresholds for rating criticism, hostility, and overinvolvement seemed to apply equally well in the early North American replications, the assessment of overinvolvement proved more challenging in some cultures. An important study in Chandigarh North India found that compared to the UK or Denmark, critical comments and overinvolvement were much less frequently rated in Chandigarh. Furthermore, in Chandigarh, city dwellers had higher levels of critical comments than village residents.[10] While the relationship between high EE and relapse was maintained, the fact that high EE was generally much less often observed in Chandigarh than in London might explain the significantly better outcome (fewer overall relapses) in Chandigarh.[11]

While suggestive of a causal role for high EE in relapse, the fundamental issue of causality can never be entirely resolved by observational studies alone. Experimental studies showing that reductions in high EE would lead to corresponding reductions of relapse were needed.

Julian's first FI study[12] recruited twenty-four recently hospitalized patients with a diagnosis of schizophrenia who lived at home with one or more family members. Eligible patients had to have had >35 hours face-to-face contact with at least one relative in their household. Relatives were then assessed for EE and those who met criteria for high EE (6 or more critical comments, any degree of hostility, or a rating of 3 or more on overinvolvement) were then randomly allocated 1:1 to receive the experimental intervention or to continue with routine outpatient care. All patients in both groups received depot antipsychotic medication. The FI included three components—education about the symptoms, course and treatments for schizophrenia; a relatives group that met every two weeks to share caring experiences, discuss problems and solutions and learn about helpful coping strategies; and finally, individual family sessions that included the patient and were carried out in the family home providing an opportunity to focus on specific issues unique to that family situation. All patients were followed up for 9 months. Relapse (the main outcome) was defined as a recurrence or substantial worsening of symptoms. In the experimental group, the intervention resulted in a marked reduction in critical comments and hostility compared to only a small reduction in the control families. Levels of overinvolvement also decreased but were small and not different between the groups. Face-to-face contact fell below 35 hours in six experimental relatives and in three control families. Over the 9 months, the relapse rate in the outpatient only control group was 50% (6/12) compared to just 9% (1/12) of patients in the experimental intervention. The trial, therefore, showed experimental evidence for the causal influence for EE but also demonstrated the effectiveness of FI.

The participants in this study were then followed up over a 2-year period.[13] Of the patients in the first trial, 7 had discontinued medication and were excluded from the follow-up in order to examine relapse among patients who continued with maintenance medication. Of the patients in the control group, 78% (7/9) relapsed in the 2-year follow-up compared with just 20% (2/10) of the patients who had received the experimental intervention.

To tease out which of the three components of the intervention were most helpful, a further study recruited patients with high contact with high-EE relatives and randomly assigned the families to education plus family therapy or to education plus a relatives only group. Eleven of the 12 families randomized to family therapy compared to only 6 of 11 families randomized to the family only group completed the intended number of sessions. The relapse rate over 9 months in the family therapy condition was 8% while that in the family only group was 17%. As before, lowing of the relapse rate was mediated by reduced EE and/or contact. At a 2-year follow-up, fewer critical comments and lower hostility were maintained while scores on overinvolvement reduced steadily throughout. The authors concluded that relatives' group should be provided in conjunction with some family sessions in the home.[14,15]

Having developed the intervention for families caring for someone suffering from schizophrenia, Julian then turned his attention to depression. As noted earlier, he had included families caring for someone suffering from depression as a comparison sample in his earlier research.[8] He noted both that most of these carers were spouses and that sensitivity to critical comments seemed to occur at a lower threshold with relapse triggered by just two critical comments recorded in the CFI. He set out to compare the relative efficacy and costs of couple therapy and antidepressant medication in the treatment and maintenance of recovery in people with depression living with a critical partner. A total of 77 patients were randomized to receive either antidepressant medication or a manualized couple therapy based on a systemic approach. Assessments at baseline, end of treatment, and follow-up included measures of depression and the partner was assessed with the CFI. Dropout was higher for drug treatment (57%) than the couple therapy (15%). Depression improved in both groups but couple therapy showed superior improvements on the Beck Depression Inventory at the end of treatment and by the end of the 2nd-year follow-up when the patients were off treatment.[16]

Community Care of Enduring Severe Mental Illness: The TAPS Program

Julian entered the field of psychiatry at a time of great change in mental healthcare. Before the second World War, many people suffering from enduring severe mental illness were incarcerated in large hospital asylums. Dissatisfaction with the costs of maintaining these old overcrowded buildings together with developments in outpatient care, the arrival of antipsychotic medication, and the launch of the NHS brought a new sense of optimism to psychiatry. In 1961, a report extrapolating from existing bed reductions suggested that asylum beds could be halved in 14 years.[17] In fact, it took some 25 years from that point to the closure of the first asylum. The early phase of asylum closure mainly involved shuffling patients between institutions and discharging the least severe to live with families or in lodging houses.

It was against this backdrop that funding was secured for a study of the outcomes of closure of Friern and Claybury Hospitals in North London. As it was not feasible or ethically appropriate to employ a randomized trial design, a method of "movers and stayers" in which successive groups of patients leaving the hospital were matched those awaiting discharge. A comprehensive battery of assessments including mental and physical health and social behavior was collected at baseline and at 1 and more years after community placement. Patients leaving hospital were accommodated in group homes in the local community with a relatively small number who because of behavioral problems moved to secure accommodation. As the discharges proceeded, there came a point at which matching the movers and stayers was no longer feasible so from this point each patient served as their own control.[18]

Summarizing the outputs of this research program that includes 48 scientific reports and a book is no easy task. Key highlights include the follow-up of 737 long-stay patients with a functional psychosis at 1 year after discharge from hospital. Of these, 24 had died (2 by suicide), 7 were lost presumed homeless, and 2 were in prison. There was very little change in symptoms or behavioral function, but patients were appreciative of the improved freedom afforded by their much less restrictive community homes. Patients' social lives were enhanced by an increase of contact with neighbors and friends though for some, there was a decrease in contact with relatives.[19] Around a third of the community patients were readmitted to hospital at some point in the follow-up. The risk of rehospitalization was greater for younger patients, those with a larger number of predischarge hospitalizations, a higher abnormal behavior score, and a history of mania.[20] Also, at the 1-year follow-up point, there were 72 long-stay patients whose behaviors were too problematic to be considered suitable for a community placement. All exhibited severe and persistent behavioral problems. These patients were placed in secure accommodation.[21]

Patients were reassessed 5 years after discharge to community settings. By this point, 126 had died largely of natural causes. Data was obtained on 523 of the survivors. There was no change in the patients' clinical symptoms or problem behaviors but patients increased domestic and community skills, acquired new friends, and the great majority wanted to remain in their current homes.[22] Looked at across the entire 13 years of the program, over 80% of long-stay patients were successfully discharged to community group homes with two-thirds still living in the residence to which they had originally been placed. There were no increases in suicide rates, only 4 patients became homeless and just 24 recorded criminal incidents of which 15 were assaults committed by 13 patients. Over the 13 years, 38% of patients were readmitted to hospital at some point of whom about a third remained in hospital for >1 year subsequently. While psychiatric symptoms and behaviors remained unchanged overall, there were gains in community skills and the majority improved quality of life. There was little difference between hospital and community costs which taken with the outcome findings suggested that community care was more effective than long-stay hospital wards.[23]

How patients were selected for placement and moved to a particular home in the community was largely a decision of hospital staff based in part on a perception of "readiness" to move and on which patients were likely to get on together in the group home settings. The earliest leavers tended to be younger, more recently hospitalized, and who were viewed as the most likely successful placements. While there was consultation with patients in working out which locations were most suitable, there was little if any consultation with the immediate neighbors of any scheme. The hospital closure program during the 1990s in England was faced by considerable resistance from the public, the press, and a few politicians in the wake of a handful of tragic events and worries about homelessness. The reticence to disclose plans to neighbors was partly to avoid expected neighborhood resistance and also on the grounds that giving such information could be a breach of the individual's right to privacy in terms of their prior psychiatric history. Julian and I teamed up to conduct a trial an experimental educational campaign focused specifically on these fears. We chose two areas in South London where patients were shortly to be placed. We carried out an attitudinal survey across both areas and then in one area conducted an educational campaign focused on the 100 or so households on either side of the proposed group home prior to the arrival of any patients. While no information about the patients was shared, the staff attending the home attended meetings to meet the neighbors, led open discussions about mental health and how care was provided and provided their contact details. The attitudinal survey was then repeated in both areas within a year of the move. While there was little achieved by way of an increase in knowledge about mental illness, there was a marked reduction of fearful and rejecting attitudes in the experimental area. Social contact with patients and staff after the move was greater and some friendships were established that endured for several years.[24]

Social Exclusion and Schizophrenia

After the second World War, Britain was very short of labor and turned to its colonies and the commonwealth to fill the gaps. Large numbers of migrants from the Indian subcontinent, parts of Africa, and the Caribbean were encouraged in their view of Britain both as an economic opportunity but also as their "mother country". But on arrival, instead of a welcoming "mother", they were met with considerable racial hostility from the white population who feared the new arrivals were taking their jobs and threatening their racial purity. Against these threats, studies among migrant communities showed a higher incidence of psychosis, higher rates of hospitalization particularly under compulsion, treatment with higher doses of medication, and fewer offers of psychotherapy particularly among black African and African-Caribbean migrants (and even among their British-born children) than their white contemporaries. Given the difference in treatment approaches, it is no wonder that the discrepancy in incidence was seen as another example of prejudice and discrimination. But what was missing in the debate was any rigorous epidemiological study of the rates between different migrant groups in Britain or of rates of psychosis in the Caribbean. To tackle this, Julian and colleagues carried out three studies in England, Trinidad, and Barbados, all three studies used similar case identification strategies and symptom assessments using the PSE and CATEGO classification system. In England, incidence rates and outcomes were examined separately for three groups of self-assigned ethnicity: Black (largely of African-Caribbean origin), Asian, and White. The Black patients had a significantly higher incidence than Whites or Asians. The African-Caribbean cases had poorer outcomes than either of the other two groups.[25] A later study explored the role of cultural identity in these participants, comparing the Asian and African-Caribbean patients with matched samples from the healthy population. The Asian patients showed close adherence to the traditional culture of the wider Asian population while the African-Caribbean patients were much less adherent to their traditional culture, showing, for example, a preference to work and live with white people that effectively reduced some of the support of their community and suggesting a causal role for marginalization.[26]

In contrast to the study in England, both Trinidad and Barbados had significantly lower incidence, resembling the rates of the white British in London.[27,28] The studies provide no definitive explanation for the excess incidence in the UK Black population but point toward differences in the social environment, including aspects of deprivation, discrimination, and social isolation.

The questions raised by these studies encouraged Julian to embark on a much larger epidemiological study in England. The AESOP (Aetiology and Ethnicity of Schizophrenia and Other Psychoses) study co-led by Sir Robin Murray set out to explore possible social and biological explanations for the ethnic differences in incidence. It used the case finding methods of the WHO ten country study and was carried out across three areas of England that had long-established African-Caribbean populations. It confirmed elevated incidence risk ratios for both African-Caribbean and Black Africans compared to the White population, particularly for schizophrenia and mania.[29] Apart from confirming the excess incidence in ethnic minorities, it is fair to say that no single factor emerged as a prime cause. Instead, the findings showed a role for multiple indicators of social disadvantage. Compared to the general population, all cases were more socially isolated and had multiple disadvantages in education, employment, housing, and relationships. Furthermore, the impact of these deprivations was cumulative with a clear linear relationship between disadvantage and odds of psychosis. While similar patterns were present across ethnicity, indices of deprivation were higher among Black Caribbean than While British subjects.[30] The other social factor that emerged strongly was separation from parents before 16 years of age. Although this risk factor also applied across ethnicity, it was more common among the Black Caribbean population.[31] The cause for the separation was not because of schizophrenia in a parent but rather that African-Caribbean parents migrating to take up employment, often left their children behind in the care of relatives, only sending for these children several years later when they had established some security. Often the children would then face parents who they had not seen for years and to other siblings born in the UK. It is possible that the disruptions in relationships and in perceptions of caring might lead to social isolation that was shown to be a risk factor for psychosis. Other hypothesized risks including exposure to racial discriminatory events and gaps in occupational expectations and achievements were not substantiated.

The AESOP study also confirmed marked differences in the pathways to care with people of African and African-Caribbean ethnicity being significantly more likely to be compulsorily hospitalized. African-Caribbean men were 3.5 times more likely than British male patients to be compulsorily admitted. Furthermore, compared with White British patients, more referrals came by a criminal justice agency with fewer referrals from family doctors, the latter being the traditional route into specialist mental health services in the UK.[32,33]

Auditory Hallucinations and AVATAR Therapy

At the very start of his research career, Julian tackled a question of susceptibility to hallucinations. He noted reports that some American prisoners of war during the Korean conflict had experienced hallucinations after exposure to "brainwashing" interrogations involving sensory deprivation and wondered if some aspects of an individual's personality might make them more susceptible. He created a simple sensory deprivation experiment using home-made equipment (a pair of obscured goggles and headphones through which he played "white noise") and recruited a group of healthy volunteers. The experiment showed that participants who had higher scores on a schizoid personality assessment were indeed susceptible.[34]

The central theme of Julian's work has always been a focus on interpersonal relationships, so it is not surprising that he should turn to considering the interaction of a patient and their verbal hallucinations as a relational affair. The clever use of simple technology to explore hallucinations at the start of his career also characterized his last scientific endeavor with an idea for a new therapy for auditory hallucinations. The idea came while thinking about a therapy approach for voices and observations of the immersive qualities of a computer game. The therapy was based on the "three-chair" approach in which patients are encouraged to enter into a dialog with a chosen voice represented by an empty chair through which dialog the patient is enabled to stand up to the voice and gain some control over it. The inspirational idea came to him that this therapy could be improved if instead of an empty chair, an interactive image representing the voice could appear on a computer screen and a dialog created in much the same way as a typical on-line web chat. The system created by his colleague Mark Huckvale at University College London achieved just this, using digital software to create an "avatar" of the entity the patient believes is talking to them and reproduces the typical sound of the voice the patients hears by using transformations of the therapist's voice. In the therapy, the patient sits in front of a screen on which the avatar appears. The therapist, sitting in another room, can talk either in their own voice or in the transformed voice of the avatar and a three-way discussion is created. Over the course of 6 sessions, the dialog is shaped by the therapist from the original hostile qualities of the voice to one conceding power and acknowledging the strength of the patient. A recording of each session is given to the patient who is encouraged to listen to it at home. In the first proof of concept study, 14 patients were randomized to receive therapy immediately and 12 to a delayed therapy group. At the end of therapy, there were substantial and highly significant reductions in hallucination scores and of the omnipotence and malevolence of the voice. The findings were replicated by the later addition of cases from the delayed therapy group. The study was remarkable in having a large and significant effect, better than that typically reported for longer courses of cognitive behavior therapy for psychosis.[35]

CURRENT RELEVANCE

The evidence from studies across >30 years since the concept of EE was first described, and showed it to be a widely replicated predictor of relapse in schizophrenia, in studies across a range of countries and cultures. Some puzzling contradictions, such as suggestions that EE only predicted relapse in men or failing to show that low EE was protective, probably reflected different approaches to measurement and study design. A meta-analysis of pooled data from 25 studies and 1,346 cases using a consistent definition of EE showed a relapse rate of 50% for those living with high-EE relatives and 21% for those with low-EE relatives. High EE was a risk for both men and women. In high-EE families, close contact additionally increased the risk of relapse while contact with low-EE relatives was protective. The benefits of residing in low-EE households and taking medication were both independently beneficial with no indication that living in a low-EE environment should influence whether medication is prescribed.[36] High-EE behaviors have also been found among care staff (e.g., in care homes) with the implication that the family approach is broadly applicable for the training of professionals, especially where they will be involved in providing long-term care.[37]

In their guidance for the NHS and wider care system in England, the National Institute for Health and Care Excellence (NICE) publishes national guidelines for the treatment of schizophrenia. This provides robust and consistent evidence that FI is effective for reducing relapse and rehospitalization and recommends that FI should be routinely available in the NHS. As in Julian's early work, the guidelines further recommend that the patient should be included in the intervention and that work with individual families is more acceptable to patients and carers than the group-based format.[38]

Given the influence of NICE and the clear recommendations, it is surprising that FI still struggles to find a home in routine care. Attempts to increase access have included making the training available to NHS professionals including nurses.[39] But sustained uptake is low even in centers where there have been robust efforts to train health staff in the therapy. Barriers to implementation include competing demands of routine work, pressures from delivery of crisis care, and significantly, a shortage of ongoing supervision after completion of training.[40] Even when these issues are addressed, sustainable long-term improvement seems difficult to achieve. A study within one large mental health provider that had been part of an intensive training initiative showed a decade later—that fewer than 10% of eligible patients and their families were offered the approach.[41]

Community care for severe mental health problems now dominates the UK. Most patients who would have ended up in the long-stay wards of the old asylum are now looked after in group living arrangements in ordinary housing stock. In the early years, the staffing of these homes came largely from the old asylums and was criticized on the grounds that they would bring with them old institutional practices. Other concerns were that the reprovision was really just transinstitutionalization, residents moving from large hospitals to a fractured system of scattered units in the community.[42] However, the staffing mix has changed over the years with more focus on staff visiting rather than residing with the patients and a clearer separation of the roles of accommodation support from the care and treatment of the mental illness. An important study of residential provision for long-term severe mental illness compared service quality, costs, and service users' quality of life across 24-hour residential care and supported housing and "floating outreach" in nationally representative regions in England. Patients in 24-hour residential care had the greatest need for care and those in floating outreach having the least, but floating outreach included fewer people with severe mental illness. Residents of supported housing were more socially included and had greater autonomy. Interestingly, quality of life was lowest among the floating outreach population perhaps reflecting the challenges of community life with less support.[43]

The way in which mental healthcare is delivered in the UK has undergone multiple reconfigurations and changes since the original hospital closures. A great deal of these changes has been attempts to improve the delivery of care outside of hospital with the introduction of multiple functional teams including early intervention, community mental healthcare teams, crisis home care, and assertive community treatment so that across the contact with mental healthcare, a patient with enduring care needs is faced with multiple changes of psychiatrist and other professionals. They may start in an early intervention team but then be handed over to a separate community team for longer-term care and see different people when in a crisis or during acute hospitalization. Julian might well say this approach flies in the face of the importance of a therapeutic relationship developed over time with a main professional carer. Indeed, our own work examining the delivery of care over a 6-year period confirms the steady decrease in continuity that correlates with poorer health outcomes.[44] Also concerning is that despite all the community reforms and rhetoric, the problems of racial biases in care that were highlighted in the AESOP study are also far from resolved. According to official NHS statistical and other data gathered to inform forthcoming changes to the Mental Health Act, black people are still over-represented in compulsory treatment settings, still more likely to be detained after contact with the criminal justice system, still less likely to be offered psychological therapies, and still more likely to report harsh or distressing experiences.[45]

In the conclusion to his book *"The Unbalanced Mind"*, Julian makes the point that despite all the knowledge we develop concerning the biological underpinnings of disorder, the future of psychiatry depends not only on these but rather on increasing understanding of relationships between people. In this respect, AVATAR therapy, that encourages the patient to enter into a dialogic relationship with their voice, has at its core the idea of a voice as a social experience. The voice is experienced as a form of communication and not simply some misattribution of internal thoughts because of some biologically based problem with cognitive self-monitoring. The findings from the first proof of principle study have now been extended and replicated in fully powered randomized controlled trials. The first of these compared 6 sessions of AVATAR therapy to supportive counseling in 150 patients with a diagnosis of schizophrenia who had heard distressing voices continuously for the previous 12 months. The finding of Julian's study was replicated and showed the therapy was safe.[46] AVATAR therapy has now been further tested in large, controlled trial run across multiple sites in the UK in which two versions of the therapy were compared to a treatment as usual control. We successfully trained >30 therapists to deliver treatment and again have had very encouraging results.[47] The next step will involve taking the therapy to routine care and testing efficacy internationally. Trials are ongoing in Canada, Denmark, and Australia but not yet reported and AVATAR therapy is shortly to be piloted in India and Ethiopia.

CONCLUDING REMARKS

Julian made a huge impact on psychiatry, particularly in the UK but also internationally. His most lasting legacy is his development of FI for psychosis that has proven effective around the world. I strongly believe this will also be the fate of AVATAR therapy.

I end this essay with a quote from my colleague Sir Robin Murray written for Julian's obituary published at King's College London. *Few psychiatrists develop any successful new treatments. Julian Leff developed four. Firstly, the value of the prophylactic use of antipsychotics to prevent the return of psychosis; secondly family therapy to reduce the adverse effects of high expressed emotion; thirdly methods of successfully returning patients to the community who had been in psychiatric hospitals for decades; and fourthly, the value of avatar therapy in reducing the voices that torment patients.*

ACKNOWLEDGMENT

I am extremely grateful to Professor Joan Raphael-Leff, for her assistance with Julian's biography and family life.

REFERENCES

1. Wing JK, Cooper JE, Sartorius N. Measurement and Classification of Psychiatric Symptoms. Cambridge: Cambridge University Press; 1974.
2. Rutter M, Brown GW. The reliability and validity of measures of family life and relationships in families containing a psychiatric patient. Soc Psychiatry. 1966;1:38-53.
3. Brown GW, Birley JL. Crises and life changes and the onset of schizophrenia. J Health Soc Behav. 1968;9:203-14.
4. Leff JP, Wing JK. Trial of maintenance therapy in schizophrenia. Br Med J. 1971;3(5775):599-604.
5. Leff JP, Hirsch SR, Gaind R, Rhode PD, Stevens BC. Life events and maintenance therapy in schizophrenic relapse. Br J Psychiatry. 1984;123:659-60.
6. Brown GW. Experiences of discharged chronic schizophrenic mental hospital patients in various types of living group. Milbank Q. 1959;37:105-31.
7. Brown GW, Birley JLT, Wing JK. Influence of family life on the course of schizophrenic disorders: a replication. Br J Psychiatry. 1972;121:241-58.
8. Leff JP, Vaughn C. The interaction of life events and relatives expressed emotion in schizophrenia and depressive neurosis. Br J Psychiatry. 1980;136:146-53.
9. Tarrier N, Vaughn C, Lader M, Leff JP. Bodily reactions to people and events in schizophrenics. Arch Gen Psychiatry. 1979;36:311-5.
10. Wig NN, Menon DK, Bedi H, Leff J, Kuipers L, Ghosh A, et al. Expressed emotion and schizophrenia in north India. II. Distribution of expressed emotion components among relatives of schizophrenic patients in Aarhus and Chandigarh. Br J Psychiatry. 1987;151:160-5. Erratum in: Br J Psychiatry. 1987;151:870.
11. Leff J, Wig NN, Ghosh A, Bedi H, Menon DK, Kuipers L, et al. Expressed emotion and schizophrenia in north India. III. Influence of relatives' expressed emotion on the course of schizophrenia in Chandigarh. Br J Psychiatry. 1987;151:166-73.

12. Leff J, Kuipers L, Berkowitz R, Eberlein-Vries R, Sturgeon D. A controlled trial of social intervention in the families of schizophrenic patients. Br J Psychiatry. 1982;141:121-34.
13. Leff J, Kuipers L, Berkowitz R, Sturgeon D. A controlled trial of social intervention in the families of schizophrenic patients: two year follow up. Br J Psychiatry. 1985;146:594-600.
14. Leff J, Berkowitz R, Shavit N, Strachan A, Glass I, Vaughn C. A trial of family therapy v. a relatives group for schizophrenia. Br J Psychiatry. 1989;154:58-66.
15. Leff J, Berkowitz R, Shavit N, Strachan A, Glass I, Vaughn C. A trial of family therapy v. a relatives group for schizophrenia: two year follow up. Br J Psychiatry. 1990;157:571-7.
16. Leff J, Vearnals S, Brewin CR, Wolff G, Alexander B, Asen E, et al. The London Depression Intervention Trial. Randomised controlled trial of antidepressants v. couple therapy in the treatment and maintenance of people with depression living with a partner: clinical outcome and costs. Br J Psychiatry. 2000;177:95-100. Erratum in: Br J Psychiatry. 2000;177:284.
17. Tooth GC, Brooke EM. Trends in the mental hospital population and their effect on future planning. Lancet. 1961;1:710-3.
18. O' Driscoll C, Leff J. The TAPS project. 9: Design of the Research Study on the long-stay patients. Br J Psychiatry. 1993;162:18-24.
19. Leff J, Trieman N, Gooch C. Team for the Assessment of Psychiatric Services (TAPS) Project 33: prospective follow-up study of long-stay patients discharged from two psychiatric hospitals. Am J Psychiatry. 1966;153:1318-24.
20. Gooch C, Leff J. Factors affecting the success of community placement: the TAPS project 26. Psychol Med. 1996;26:511-20.
21. Trieman N, Leff J. The TAPS project. 36: the most difficult to place long-stay psychiatric in-patients. Outcome one year after relocation. Team for the Assessment of Psychiatric Services. Br J Psychiatry. 1996;169:289-92.
22. Leff J, Treiman N. Long-stay patients discharged from psychiatric hospitals. Social and clinical outcomes after five years in the community. TAPS Project 46. Br J Psychiatry. 2000;174:217-23.
23. Leff J, Treiman N, Knapp M, Hallam A. The TAPS Project. A report on 13 years of research, 1985–1998. Psychiatr Bull. 2000;24:165-8.
24. Wolff G, Pathare S, Craig T, Leff J. Public education for community care: a new approach. Br J Psychiatry. 1996;168:441-7.
25. Bhugra D, Leff J, Mallett R, Der G, Corridan B, Rudge S. Incidence and outcome of schizophrenia in Whites, African-Caribbeans and Asians in London. Psychol Med. 1997;27:791-8.
26. Bhugra D, Leff J, Mallett R, Morgan C, Zhao JH. The culture and identity schedule. A measure of cultural affiliation: acculturation, marginalization and schizophrenia. Int J Soc Psychiatry. 2010;56:540-56.
27. Bhugra D, Hilwig M, Hossein B, Marceau H, Neehall J, Leff J, et al. First-contact incidence rates of schizophrenia in Trinidad and one-year follow-up. Br J Psychiatry. 1996;169:587-92.
28. Mahy GE, Mallett R, Leff J, Bhugra D. First-contact incidence rate of schizophrenia on Barbados. Br J Psychiatry. 1999;175:28-33.
29. Fearon P, Kirkbride JB, Morgan C, Dazzan P, Morgan K, Lloyd T, et al. Incidence of schizophrenia and other psychoses in ethnic minority groups: results from the MRC AESOP study. Psychol Med. 2006;36:1541-60.

30. Morgan C, Kirkbride J, Hutchinson G, Craig T, Morgan K, Dazzan P, et al. Cumulative social disadvantage, ethnicity and first-episode psychosis: a case-control study. Psychol Med. 2008;38:1701-15.
31. Morgan C, Kirkbride J, Leff J, Craig T, Hutchinson G, McKenzie K, et al. Parental separation, loss and psychosis in different ethnic groups: A case-control study. Psychol Med. 2007;37:495-503.
32. Morgan C, Mallett R, Hutchinson G, Bagalkote H, Morgan K, Fearon P, et al. Pathways to carte and ethnicity 1: sample characteristics and compulsory admission. Br J Psychiatry. 2005;186:281-9.
33. Morgan C, Mallett R, Hutchinson G, Bagalkote H, Morgan K, Fearon P, et al. Pathways to care and ethnicity. 2: source of referral and help seeking. Br J Psychiatry. 2005;184:290-6.
34. Leff JP. Perceptual phenomena and personality in sensory deprivation. Br J Psychiatry. 1968;114:1499-508.
35. Leff J, Williams G, Huckvale MA, Arbuthnot M, Leff AP. Computer-assisted therapy for medication-resistant auditory hallucinations: proof-of-concept study. Br J Psychiatry. 2013;202:428-33.
36. Bebbington P, Kuipers L. The predictive utility of expressed emotion in schizophrenia: an aggregate analysis. Psychol Med. 1994;24:707-19.
37. Ball A, Moor E, Kuipers L. Expressed emotion in community care staff. A comparison of patient outcome in a nine-month follow-up of two hostels. Soc Psychiatry Psychiatr Epidemiol. 1992;27:35-9.
38. National Institute for Health and Care Excellence. (2014). NICE Guideline: Psychosis and Schizophrenia in Adults: Prevention and management. [online] Available from www.nice.org.uk/guidance/cg178. [Last accessed February, 2025]
39. Leff J, Sharpley M, Chisholm D, Bell R, Gamble C. Training community psychiatric nurses in schizophrenia family work: a study of clinical and economic outcomes for patients and relatives. J Ment Health. 2001;10:189-97.
40. Berry K, Haddock G. The implementation of the NICE guidelines for schizophrenia: barriers to the implementation of psychological interventions and recommendations for the future. Psychol Psychother. 2008;81:419-36.
41. Prytys M, Garety P, Jolley S, Onwumere J, Craig T. Implementing the NICE guideline for schizophrenia recommendations for psychological therapies: a qualitative analysis of the attitudes of CMHT staff. Clin Psychol Psychother. 2011;18:48-59.
42. Priebe S, Badesconyi A, Fioritti A, Hansson L, Kilian R, Torres-Gonzales F, et al. Reinstitutionalisation in mental health care: comparison of data on service provision from six European countries. Br Med J. 2005;330(7483):123-6.
43. Killaspy H, Marston L, Green N, Harrison I, Lean M, Holloway F, et al. Clinical outcomes and costs for people with complex psychosis; a naturalistic prospective cohort study of mental health rehabilitation service users in England. BMC Psychiatry. 2016;16:95.
44. Macdonald A, Adams D, Craig T, Murray R. Continuity of care and clinical outcomes in the community for people with severe mental illness. Br J Psychiatry. 2019;214:273-8.

45. Parliament UK. (2022). Mental Health Act Reform - Race and Ethnic Inequalities. [online] Available from https://researchbriefings.files.parliament.uk/documents/POST-PN-0671/POST-PN-0671.pdf. [Last accessed February, 2025]
46. Craig T, Rus-Calafell M, Ward T, Leff JP, Huckvale M, Howarth E, et al. AVATAR therapy for auditory verbal hallucinations in people with psychosis: a single-blind, randomised controlled trial. Lancet Psychiatry. 2018;5:31-40.
47. Garety PA, Edwards CJ, Jafari H, Emsley R, Huckvale M, Rus-Calafell M, et al. Digital AVATAR therapy for distressing voices in psychosis: the phase 2/3 AVATAR2 trial. Nat Med. 2024;30(12):3658-68. https://doi.org/10.1038/s41591-024-03252-8.

Appendix

Appendix

A VENKOBA RAO

Roy A Kallivayalil

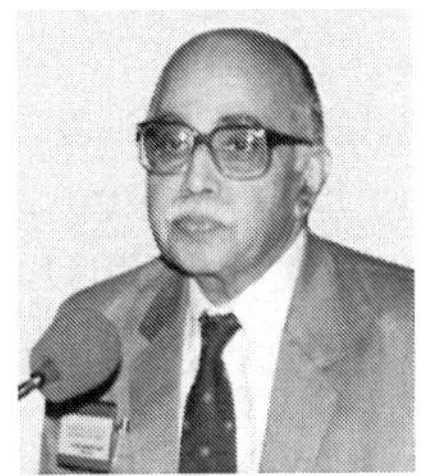

(1927–2005)

Known for his pioneering research contribution to psychiatry in India, Antapur Venkoba Rao was born in the village Kavuttalam, Andhra Pradesh. A great teacher and an inspiring speaker, he received his PhD and DSc degrees from the University of Madras. He was Chairman of the Institute of Psychiatry, Madurai Medical College, for 23 years and later Emeritus Professor and officer-in-charge of the Indian Council of Medical Research Advanced Centre on "Health and Behavior," at Madurai Medical College from 1986 to 1993. He had over 400 publications and many books authored or edited by him, including *Psychiatry of Old Age in India, Depression and Suicide Behavior, Textbook of Psychiatry, Culture, Philosophy,* and *Mental Health* and *Mind: Turbulent and Tranquil.* He was President of the Indian Psychiatric Society, founder President of the Indian Association for Social Psychiatry, and Editor of the *Indian Journal of Psychiatry (1970–78).* He was recipient of the Dr. B.C. Roy National Award, Tirumurti Lecture Award from the Indian National Science Academy, D.L.N. Murthi Rao Oration Award and J.C. Marfatia Award from the Indian Psychiatric Society, and N.N. De Oration Award. He traveled widely and was known internationally. He was visiting scientist (Fogarty) at the National Institute of Mental Health, Bethesda, USA, in 1986. He was a Fellow of the National Academy of Medical Sciences (India) and the Indian Science Academy. His chief interests were depressive disorders, psychiatry of old age, suicidology, transcultural psychiatry, and history of psychiatry. As chief investigator of the ICMR project on the aged, he evolved a model of healthcare delivery to the rural aged in India. He also pioneered geriatric psychiatry research in India. He also interpreted and incorporated India's scriptures and ancient philosophies into contemporary mental health concepts. He was well known for his lectures and writings on the Bhagavad Gita and its implications for psychiatry.

ALAN FLISHER

David Ndetei, Roy A Kallivayalil

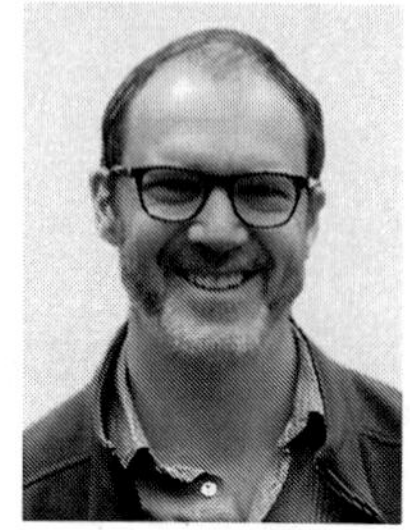
(1957–2010)

One of the most gifted and influential South African child and adolescent psychiatrists, Alan Flisher was born in Cape Town in1957 and died untimely in 2010, aged 53 years. Besides being an adviser to the South African Government and to the World Health Organization (WHO), he was also one of the founders of the Movement for Global Mental Health. He began not as a psychiatrist but as a psychologist practicing for 6 years before going on to train in medicine. He became Director of the Division of Child and Adolescent Psychiatry at the University of Cape Town in 2003 and from 2007 he served there as the Sue Streungmann Chair of Child and Adolescent Psychiatry and Mental Health. With over 200 peer-reviewed articles and 70 books or book chapters, his extensive research substantially advanced the field of public mental health in South Africa. His collaboration with the Department of Health and WHO resulted in the creation of evidence-based guidelines, standards for mental health services, and assessments of public mental health initiatives. His expertise in suicide epidemiology and prevention established vital research collaborations linking substance abuse, HIV prevention, and mental health, particularly among adolescents. His dedication extended internationally, collaborating on child and adolescent psychiatry education in Tanzania and Kenya, and leading a multicountry study that developed mental health policy in South Africa, Ghana, Zambia, and Uganda. Flisher's commitment to social justice was evident throughout his career, reflected in his active involvement in antiapartheid mental health organizations and his focus on the needs of marginalized youth and children. Flisher's legacy is characterized by integrity, compassion, and a profound commitment to enlightening mental health care and outcomes for the most marginalized populations.

dmndetei@amhf.or.ke
roykalli@gmail.com

ANGEL OTERO

Juan E Mezzich, Roy A Kallivayalil

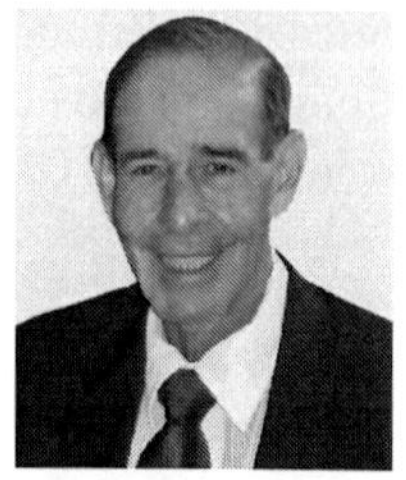
(1940–2016)

Ángel Arturo Otero Ojeda (1940–2016) unfolded his career fully in Cuba, as a Professor at the University of La Habana. He had close interactions with eminent psychiatrists from all over the world who were attracted by his creativity and solid academic contributions. He distinguished himself also as a musician and poet. He was a long-time editor of the seminal Journal of the Hospital Psiquiatrico de La Habana. His magnus opus was the Third Cuban Glossary of Psychiatry, which following on the steps of his mentor and editor of the first edition of this work, Professor Carlos Acosta Nodal, intended to adapt the International Classification of Diseases to the reality and needs of the Cuban population. They characteristically constructed these adaptations through painstaking and consensus-seeking seminars, starting with local and progressing toward national instances along all the Cuban territory with the participation of representatives of all mental health professions. Its innovative multiaxial structure articulates clinical disorders, dysfunctions, environmental factors, and psychopathogenic factors. He represented Cuba at international scientific events, where he stood out for the professionalism that characterized him and the ethical-humanistic approach that he gave to each of his presentations and interventions. Otero's indefatigable efforts to serve human beings and communities in Cuba and across the world through integral care and health promotion are consonant with verses of his preferred poet, Jose Marti, who said *if I served before now, I do not remember. What I want is to serve more.*

juanmezzich@aol.com
roykalli@gmail.com

ARTHUR MICHAEL KLEINMAN

Rama Rao Gogineni

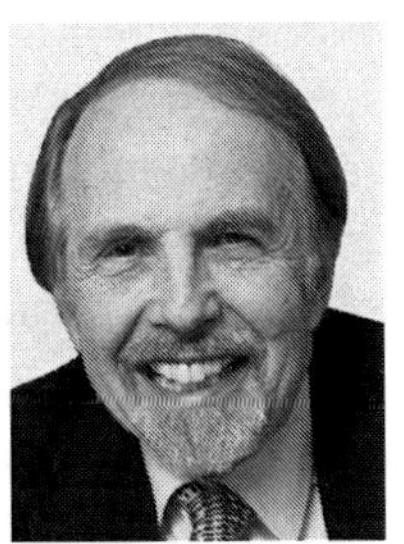
(Born - 1941)

Arthur Kleinman was born on March 1, 1941, in Lawrence, Ohio. He was married to the late Joan Kleinman (who died in 2011) for 45 years and fathered Peter and Anne. He is an American psychiatrist, social anthropologist, and a professor of medical anthropology, psychiatry, and global health and social medicine at Harvard University. Arthur Kleinman received MD from Stanford University, MA in Social Anthropology from Harvard, and psychiatric residency at the Massachusetts General Hospital. His areas of expertise include medical anthropology, cultural psychiatry, global health, social medicine, medical humanities, and China studies. Kleinman has taught for decades, supervised and mentored undergraduate students, anthropology graduate students, medical students, and postdoctoral fellows.

Kleinman has authored seven books and over 350 articles, book chapters, reviews, and introductions. Perhaps Kleinman's most influential work is *Patients and Healers in the Context of Culture* (1980), followed by *The Illness Narratives: Suffering, Healing, and the Human Condition* (1988) and *Social Origins of Distress and Disease: Depression, Neurasthenia, and Pain in Modern China* (1986), *What Really Matters* (2006), and *The Soul of Care: The Moral Education of a Husband and a Doctor* (2019). He has co-authored *A Passion for Society: How We Think About Human Suffering* (2016), *Deep China: The Moral Life of the Person. What Anthropology and Psychiatry Tell Us about*

China Today (2011). He is co-editor of 29 volumes, including: *Social Suffering, Culture and Depression, SARS in China, Global Pharmaceuticals, Subjectivity: Ethnographic Investigations, Reimagining Global Health: An Introduction, The Culture of Illness and Psychiatric Practice in Africa,* and *The Ground Between: Anthropologists Engage Philosophy* and 11 special issues of journals and published essays in *The Lancet, New England Journal of Medicine,* and *The Harvard Magazine.* Kleinman has been the recipient of many awards, prizes, and named lectureships. He is considered by many as teacher and mentor in all areas of his expertise.

ASSEN V JABLENSKY

Mohan Isaac

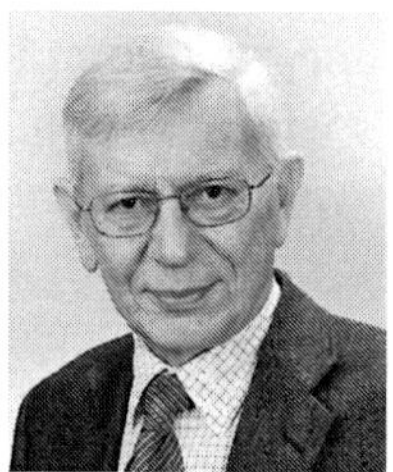

(1940–2024)

Assen Vehiaminov Jablensky was born in and completed his medical studies and training in psychiatry in Sofia, Bulgaria. Because of his excellent English, as a young psychiatrist in a mental hospital, Assen had the opportunity to act as a translator for Professor Michael Shepherd who came to Bulgaria to lecture. Shepherd offered Assen a position as his registrar at the Maudsley Hospital and Institute of Psychiatry in London where he spent 2 significant years. His close relationship with Professor Shepherd was very influential in Assen's life. Assen spent very productive 12 years (1975-1987) with the World Health Organization in Geneva where he was able to make outstanding contributions to psychiatric epidemiology, nosology, and transcultural psychiatry. Assen was the Principal Investigator of the successor of the "International Pilot Study of Schizophrenia", the influential *WHO* Ten-Country Study of Schizophrenia in different cultures ("Determinants of Outcome of Severe Mental Disorders" study which showed that the outcome of schizophrenia was significantly better in developing countries such as India and Nigeria than in developed countries such as USA and UK)—and the Collaborative Study on Depressive Disorders in Different Cultures. Assen also chaired the WHO Task Force which developed the ICD-10 classification and diagnostic guidelines for mental and behavioral disorders. Assen moved to Perth, Australia, to take up the Chair of Psychiatry at the University of Western Australia in 1993 where he worked until his retirement and established one of the strongest, research-intensive departments of psychiatry in Australia. He was the Chief Investigator of the influential large population-based study of persons living with psychotic illness—Australian National Survey of High Impact Psychosis. For his outstanding contributions, Assen received numerous awards including Eric Stromgren Prize for Psychiatric Epidemiology, Hermann Simon Prize for Social Psychiatry, and Founders Medal from the Australian Society for Psychiatric Research.

AUBREY LEWIS

Mohan Isaac

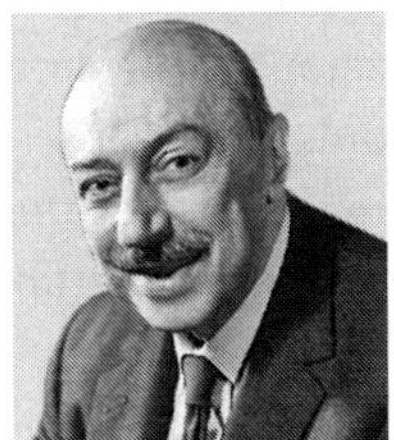
(1900–1975)

Born in Adelaide, South Australia, Aubrey Julian Lewis completed his medical studies at the University of Adelaide with distinction. As a registrar at the Royal Adelaide Hospital, Aubrey undertook anthropological research on aborigines. A Rockefeller Foundation fellowship in psychological medicine helped Aubrey to train under the mentorship of Adolf Meyer—a lasting influence on his future life and work—at the famous Phipps Clinic at John Hopkins in USA and under Karl Bonhoeffer in Berlin. After 2 years of postgraduate study, Aubrey Lewis joined the staff of the Maudsley Hospital in London in 1928 and became its Clinical Director in 1936. In 1946, the hospital was designated the Institute of Psychiatry under the auspices of the University of London. Aubrey Lewis was appointed the inaugural Chair of psychiatry—a position he held until his retirement in 1966. Through his intellect and remarkable qualities as a teacher, clinician, researcher, writer, administrator, and leader, Aubrey molded the Institute of Psychiatry into a model of scientific research and teaching in all aspects of mental health. He was able to attract the best and the brightest medical graduates to the institute and through his great scholarship, and inspirational qualities, guided and mentored future world leaders of psychiatry such as Sir Martin Roth, Michael Shepperd, Sir Michael Rutter, and Sir David Goldberg. The work of Institute of Psychiatry under the leadership of Aubrey Lewis helped to raise the status and profile of psychiatry worldwide. Aubrey Lewis started and directed the Medical Research Council Social Psychiatry Unit until his retirement. Aubrey's collected papers on psychiatric topics were edited and published by his students in three volumes—Inquiries in Psychiatry, The State of Psychiatry, and The Later Papers of Sir Aubrey Lewis. He also wrote several hundred book reviews. Aubrey was knighted in 1959.

FREDERICK REDLICH

Salman Akhtar

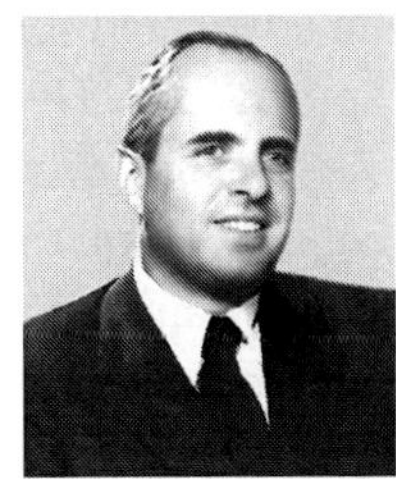
(1910–2004)

Frederick Carl Redlich was a Vienna-born North American emigre psychiatrist who chaired the Department of Psychiatry at Yale University (1950–1957) and later became the Dean of its School of Medicine. He was a recipient of Distinguished Service Awards from the American Psychiatric Association and the American College of Psychiatrists. Fritz Redlich (as he was generally called) became renowned with his 1959s' investigation of the relationship between mental illness and socioeconomic class. Conducted in collaboration with the prominent sociologist August Hollingshead, the Hollingshead-Redlich Study (as it came to be known) was marked by an astoundingly large sample of subjects and by its meticulous correlation not only of diagnoses but also of treatment modalities with social class. Its results revealed that those belonging to upper classes were less often diagnosed schizophrenic and more often treated with psychotherapy in private settings. Individuals from lower socioeconomic strata received the psychotic label more often and were subjected more frequently to bodily intrusive (e.g., ECT) interventions. This pioneering study is credited with contributing to the advent of "social psychiatry" as a subspecialty and with the establishment of community mental health centers, a few years later, in the United States. Redlich, who also authored a highly acclaimed biography of Adolf Hitler (1998), was celebrated outside of organized psychiatry as well, being elected to be a member of the American Academy of Arts and Sciences.

GEORGE VASSILIOU

George M Gournas, George Christodoulou

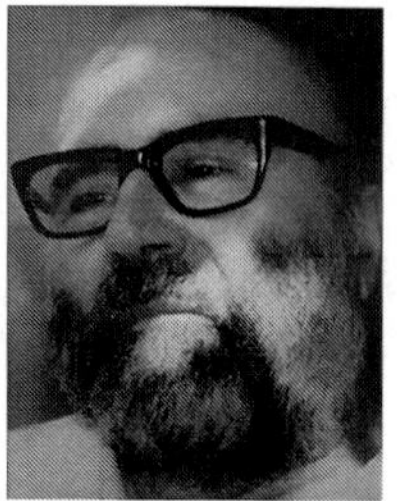

(1927–2001)

George Vassiliou, a Greek psychiatrist, was a key figure in the development of social psychiatry. In 1963, with his wife psychologist Vasso Vassiliou, he founded the Athenian Institute of Anthropos (AIA), a leading center for the development of systemic approaches to mental health. With their associates, they advanced the *systemic approach to mental health* by focusing on how individuals, families, and groups function as interconnected systems within their sociocultural environments and by orienting therapy to address relationships rather than individuals.

Vassiliou's approach to therapy, deeply rooted in *General Systems Theory*, shaped the AIA "Systemic-Dialectic Multilevel-Multifocal Approach", a comprehensive model emphasizing the fluid, evolving relationships between individuals and the social structures. A dedicated researcher on how "subjective culture" and societal changes impact families and groups, he advocated for the importance of tailoring "milieu-specific" therapeutic approaches. He developed the innovative "Synallactic Collective Image Technique," which promotes healing by helping group members reflect collectively on their personal experiences and emotions through drawing.

A strong advocate for preventive mental health, he emphasized the need for cooperative dialogue among professionals to serve Anthropos, the "whole human being".

Vassiliou's pivotal role in several professional organizations such as the World Association of Social Psychiatry (President, 1978–1983) and the Mediterranean Association for Social Psychiatry (founder, 1972) helped build an international network of professionals committed to addressing the complexities of modern societies. He trained therapists at multiple centers, academies, and associations across the world, as the American Association of Group Psychotherapy and the European Family Therapy Association, being awarded certificates in recognition of his contribution.

Vassiliou's legacy is his holistic systemic vision of mental health, prioritizing culturally relevant, family, group, and community-based approaches that focus on people's relationships and their environment in a personally meaningful and socially useful way.

JAVIER MARIATEGUI

Juan E Mezzich, Roy A Kallivayalil

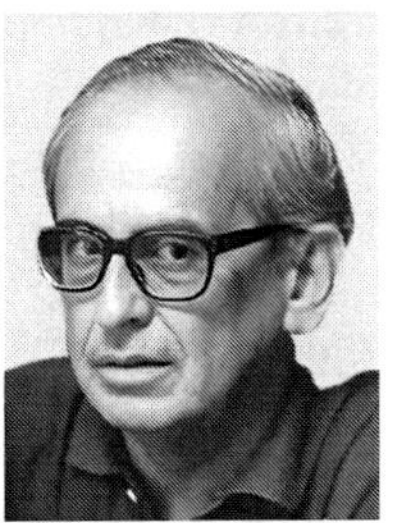

(1928–2008)

Javier Mariátegui Chiappe was a renowned Peruvian intellectual, psychiatrist, and academician. He was the last son of the arguably most important thinker on and discussant of national life, Jose Carlos Mariategui, *el Amauta*, author of *Seven Essays of Interpretation of Peruvian Reality.* He *studied at the* University of San Marcos *where he also started teaching; he was also a founder of* Cayetano Heredia University. Javier Mariategui devoted part of his life to cultivating and promoting the ideas of his admired father. The broad range of his interests and talents is illustrated, first, by his highly praised medical graduation thesis, *Psychopathology of the Experimental Intoxication with the Diethylamide of the d-Lysergic Acid.* Later, he was senior editor of the seminal *Studies of Social Psychiatry in Peru, Psychiatric Epidemiology of an Urban District in Lima, Studies of Psychiatric Epidemiology in Latin America,* and *Socio-Psychiatry in Peru.* He also became a preferred disciple of the most famous Peruvian psychiatrist of his time, Honorio Delgado. In the last period of his productive life, Mariategui became Founder and Director of the Honorio Delgado-Hideyo Noguchi National Institute of Mental Health in Lima. His intellectual work in the field of psychiatry and humanities made him a Member of the National Medicine Academy (1987) and of Peruvian Academy of the Language (1993). In 1994 he became Professor Emeritus of the Medicine Faculty of the University of San Marcos and in 1999 of the Peruvian University Cayetano Heredia.

juanmezzich@aol.com
roykalli@gmail.com

JUAN MARCONI TASSARA

Fernando Lolas Stepke

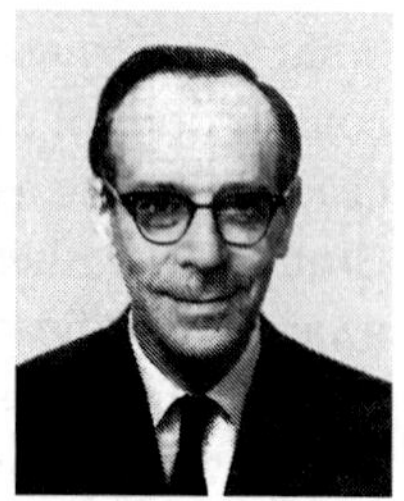
(1924–2005)

Juan Marconi was born in Valparaíso, Chile, on March 6, 1924. In Santiago, he studied at the Alonso de Ercilla Institute and entered the Faculty of Medicine at the Catholic University and later at the University of Chile, graduating in 1948. As a student, Juan Marconi joined the Institute for Research on Alcoholism founded in 1950, directed by the professor of pharmacology at the University of Chile, Jorge Mardones Restat, where work was done on two levels: Basic research and clinical and epidemiological research. There he carried out a notable academic activity and made numerous publications, recognizing that this experience was the germ of his later development in the epidemiological approach in mental health and clinical psychiatry. In 1992, Marconi received the title of Master of Chilean Psychiatry from the Society of Neurology, Psychiatry, and Neurosurgery and was honored as an important figure in Latin American Psychiatry at the XIX Latin American Congress of Psychiatry in Mar del Plata in 1997. In 2002, at the age of 78 years, he retired from the University of Chile after 52 years of practicing the profession, moving with his family to Villarrica where he died on November 17, 2005. Between 1968 and 1973, a psychiatric reform was attempted in a restricted area of Santiago in parallel with the revolutionary sociopolitical changes experienced in the country. A central figure in this movement was Juan Marconi, who went from being a university researcher to becoming the leader and promoter of a radical change in psychiatric care and mental health. He developed a model of intervention with community participation in important health problems such as alcoholism, neurosis, and sensory deprivation which benefited the population. Juan Marconi's contributions to psychiatry and mental health, although criticized from the beginning and interrupted after the military coup, significantly influenced mental health care in Chile once democracy was restored.

JULIO ARBOLEDA-FLÓREZ

Heather Stuart, Roy A Kallivayalil

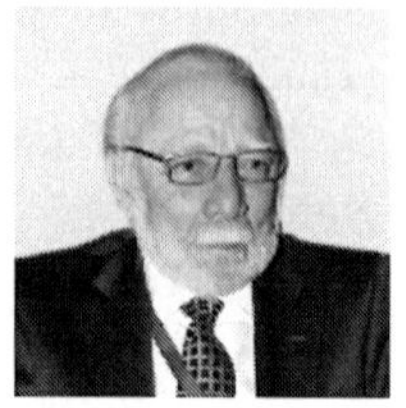
(1939–2020)

Julio Arboleda-Flórez was born in Colombia and graduated with a degree in medicine from the Universidad Nacional of Colombia in Bogota before he came to Canada to study psychiatry. He graduated in psychiatry at the University of Ottawa and went on to study forensic psychiatry at the University of Toronto. He studied epidemiology at The University of Calgary and graduated with a PhD, making him the only forensic psychiatric epidemiologist in the world. He held many distinguished positions in hospitals, correctional facilities, and universities and was active in the World Psychiatric Association, the World Association of Social Psychiatry, the International Academy of Law and Mental Health, and the World Health Organization, where he directed a regional unit for research and training in psychiatric epidemiology. Throughout his career, he made pioneering contributions to the scholarly literature in law, psychiatric epidemiology, psychiatric ethics, forensic psychiatry, and social psychiatry. He received numerous awards and recognitions from medical and scientific societies in Canada and elsewhere. He was fluent in many languages, including Latin, and a generous supporter of young researchers in lower- and middle-income countries, where he mentored many residents and students throughout his career. Working with colleagues from the World Psychiatric Association, he was instrumental in developing and evaluating global antistigma activities directed toward people with schizophrenia—work that subsequently informed a 20 plus country roll-out of the World Psychiatric Association's global program to fight the stigma associated with schizophrenia. He served as the President of the World Association for Social Psychiatry during 2007–2010 during which he made sustained efforts to promote social psychiatry in the low- and middle-income (LAMI) countries. He was an avid reader and traveler with a disarming sense of humor and infectious laugh. He was a sought-after colleague, friend, and mentor.

SUDHIR KAKAR

Salman Akhtar

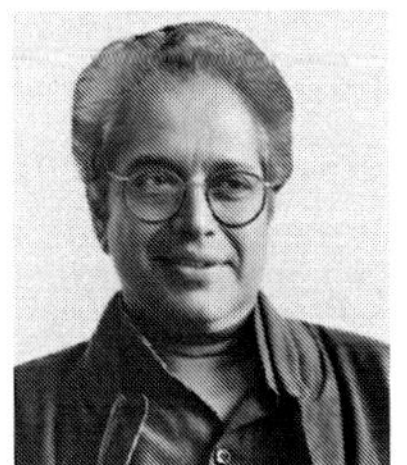
(1938–2024)

Mentored by the great socioculturally oriented psychoanalyst Erik Erikson (on whose life and work this book contains a full chapter) and trained in psychoanalysis in Frankfurt, Germany, Sudhir Kakar was a somewhat late arrival on the scene of culturally suffused clinical thought. He had dabbled in mechanical engineering, macroeconomics, and short story writing before he embarked on a career in "anthropological psychoanalysis'" While he still made occasional forays in spirituality, historical fiction, and mysticism, his better known and lasting contributions remained in the field of culturally informed depth psychology. Distressed by the sharp elbows of the Eurocentrism that pervaded early psychoanalysis, Kakar produced a large body of work that explicated child development, personality functioning, and sexuality in terms of Indian culture. His seminal books *The Inner World* (1978) and *Intimate Relations* (1990) opened up new vistas in the understanding of affective and erotic life of the people of India. Kakar soon gained international recognition. He taught at Harvard and Columbia Universities in the United States, collaborated with masterful (though controversial) Indologist Wendy Donninger, and received numerous awards, including Germany's Goethe Prize for Literature, an honor that had been bestowed upon only one other psychoanalyst before him and that analyst was none other than Sigmund Freud. Kakar's collected works appeared under the title of *The Essential Writings of Sudhir Kakar, Volumes I–V* (2024), a few months after his death. His inclusion here is a reflection of the great impact he has had on the culturally attuned formulations of psychotherapists in India as well as an expression of the hope that psychiatric trainees and practicing psychiatrists in India shall also partake of his vast and deep creative output.

TSUTOMU SAKUTA

Roy A Kallivayali

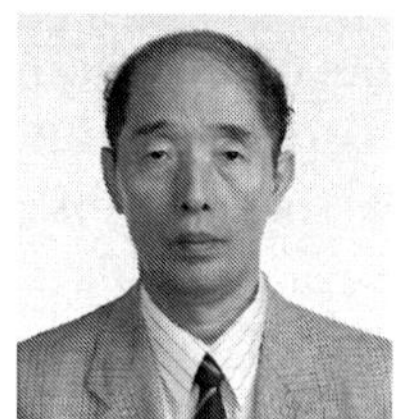
(1943–2020)

Professor Tsutomu Sakuta was born in Tokyo, Japan, on June 25, 1943. In 1968, he graduated from Keio University Faculty of Medicine in Tokyo, Department of Neuropsychiatry, with an MD and then a PhD. His main interest was in forensic psychiatry (social aspects of delinquency among adolescents, infanticide, prison psychiatry in Japan, personality, and fostering). In 1994, he received the International Council Prison Medical Services Special award. His article on "Constitutional and organizational elements of forensic psychiatry in Japan", published in the Current Opinion in Psychiatry (2003), was a landmark. He was President of the World Association for Social Psychiatry (2003–2007) and also a member of the board of the International Federation for Psychotherapy and the International Academy of Law and Mental Health. He actively promoted international collaboration between countries for peace. He was the president of the Japan International Cultural Exchange Foundation whose purpose was "to improve human culture and promote world peace through various international cultural exchange activities." He put this to practice by generously contributing to Early Career Psychiatrists Fellowships at the World Congresses of Social Psychiatry in Marrakech (2010), Lisbon (2013), New Delhi (2016), and Bucharest (2019) and serving as a mentor to the early career psychiatrists. Sakuta was a creative educationalist and founded the Japan University of Health Sciences. His commitment to social psychiatry, international peace, and scientific collaborations will ever be remembered.

VIDYA SAGAR

Savita Malhotra, Roy A Kallivayalil

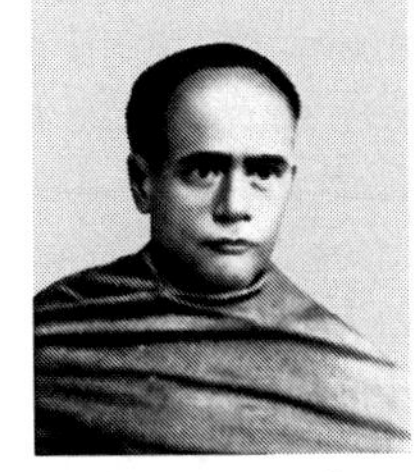
(1909–1978)

Vidya Sagar Diwan is a legendary figure in Indian psychiatry who had dedicated his life to the service of the people, first in the state of undivided Panjab and later in Haryana, India. After getting his membership of the Royal College of Psychiatrists (MRCP) from the Institute of Psychiatry in London (1948–1951), he joined as the Superintendent of the Panjab Mental Hospital Amritsar (1951–1966) and shifted to Rohtak Medical College as the Head, Department of Psychiatry, in 1966. He was the founder member of the Royal College of Social Psychiatry (1974) and the President of the Indian Psychiatric Society in 1973. Dr Vidya Sagar had great wisdom and pragmatism in aligning the systems of mental health care with the sociocultural ethos prevalent in India. He emphasized on the need to involve family in treatment of the mentally ill, keeping the patient at ease and family integrated. This was quite in contrast to the then prevailing system of psychiatric care being provided in mental hospitals where patients are separated from the family for variable periods of time and invariably are abandoned by the family. He started training programs in psychiatry for medical students, nurses, schoolteachers, social workers, and probationary officers working in various settings like medical colleges, schools, and remand homes, thus integrating psychiatry in other medical specialties, popularizing it in the community and helping to reduce stigma. He believed that persons with mental illness needed to be integrated back in society after treatment and the social institutions must come forward to make them active members of the society again. Vidya Sagar was the most renowned social psychiatrist of his times, a humanist, full of compassion for the mentally ill and their families, a selfless man, revered by his patients. He was ahead of his times in propagating family psychiatry, community psychiatry, psychoeducation, and mass psychotherapy, in times when psychiatry was primarily practiced in mental hospitals.

WOLFGANG RUTZ

Roy A Kallivayalil, Marianne C Kastrup

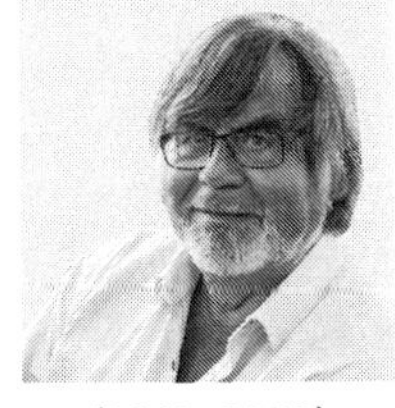
(1943–2023)

After his training as a medical doctor and a psychiatrist in Germany and Austria, Wolfgang Rutz, since 1970, had worked in Sweden, holding positions at the Karolinska and Uppsala Universities. An important part of his career took place on the Swedish island, Gotland, where he was responsible for mental health services. From 1998 to 2004, he was the Regional Officer for Mental Health, at the WHO

Europe. Further, he was a professor of social psychiatry at the University of Applied Sciences, Coburg, Germany. In 1983–1984, the Swedish Committee for the Prevention and Treatment of Depression introduced an educational program for all general practitioners (GPs) in Gotland. The primary goal was to increase knowledge about the diagnosis and treatment of patients with affective disorders. The study was scientifically evaluated and became later internationally known as the "Gotland Study" under the leadership of Wolfgang Rutz. The educational program led to a dramatic decrease in depression-related morbidity and mortality on the island. Especially noted were the rates of suicide that, before the educational intervention, were the highest in Sweden; these dropped down to the lowest figures, primarily in females. The results of the Gotland study have provided evidence for the view that early recognition and adequate treatment of depression are essential methods of suicide prevention. During the period of European transition, he wrote about how societal stress and loss of social cohesion and spiritual values have affected morbidity and mortality. He said that the stress of societal transition had taken its toll among indigenous people in Greenland, farmers in Ireland, and also in Eastern Europe, where figures for the main causes of illness and death often greatly exceeded those of neighboring populations. He was Co-chair of the World Association of Social Psychiatry Section on migration and mental health since 2019. He brought public health perspective and the social determinants of mental health into discourse repeatedly. This was one of his lasting contributions.

roykalli@gmail.com
d121304@dadlnet.dk

Index